WALKING FOR FITNESS
THE BEGINNER'S HANDBOOK

WALKING

FOR FITNESS

THE BEGINNER'S HANDBOOK

MARNIE CARON
& THE SPORT MEDICINE COUNCIL
OF BRITISH COLUMBIA

GREYSTONE BOOKS

Douglas & McIntyre Publishing Group

Vancouver/Toronto/Berkeley

Greystone Books
A division of Douglas & McIntyre Ltd.
2323 Quebec Street, Suite 201
Vancouver, British Columbia
Canada V5T 4S7
www.greystonebooks.com

Library and Archives Canada Cataloguing in Publication
Caron, Marnie
Walking for fitness : the beginner's handbook / Marnie Caron and the
Sport Medicine Council of British Columbia.
Includes index.
ISBN 978-1-55365-219-9
1. Fitness walking. I. Sport Medicine Council of B.C. II. Title.
RA781.65.C38 2007   613.7'176   C2006-905604-8

Editing by Lucy Kenward
Cover design by Naomi MacDougall
Text design by Warren Clark
Cover photography courtesy of First Light
Printed and bound in Canada by Friesens
Printed on acid-free paper
Distributed in the U.S. by Publishers Group West

We gratefully acknowledge the financial support of the Canada Council for the Arts, the British Columbia Arts Council, and the Government of Canada through the Book Publishing Industry Development Program (BPIDP) for our publishing activities.

This book is dedicated
to my grandmothers
whose strength and wisdom
made my journey easier:
Georgina Lyle and
Stanzel Trawick.

Contents

Acknowledgments

I would like to thank the following friends and colleagues for your support, guidance and expertise in putting this project together: Dr. Bryan Barootes, Dr. Jim Bovard, Lynda Cannell, Dr. Diane Finegood, Sandy Friedman, Jennifer Gibson, Dr. Liz Joy, Lynn Kanuka, Lucy Kenward, Jill Lambert, Dr. Teresa Liu-Ambrose, Thom Lutes, Brad Moore, Phil Moore, Diana Rochon, Dr. Whitney Sedgwick and Dr. Trent Smith.

Foreword

SOMETIMES, WHEN I'M FOLDING THE LAUNDRY OR DOING the dishes, I ask myself: "Did I really stand on the Olympic podium and receive a bronze medal for myself and for Canada?" As long ago as that moment was, the answer is, of course, "You bet I did!" For a little 5-foot-nothing runner from Saskatchewan, it really was a dream come true.

These days, I no longer train or compete, and the only running I do is to keep up with my four kids! However, through my work as InTraining Program Director at the Sport Medicine Council of British Columbia, my passion for fitness has been revitalized as I find myself able to share my expertise with people like you, who for your own reasons have decided you'd like to become more active. Even though at this moment you may be a little unsure of yourself, I know that with proper guidance you will discover how simple starting to exercise can be and how it will make such a difference in your life. On a personal level, it's been wonderful to be able to help people find an exercise path that is right for them: I had no idea of the tremendous strength and inspiration I would receive from those who truly take charge of their personal goals for fitness and then discover the joy in their accomplishments.

Congratulations to you! You've already begun your new lifestyle, because you've made the decision that your health is important to you and you've started to read this book. *Walking for Fitness* will guide you with expert advice, tips and encouragement from people just like you who have improved their health, managed their weight, overcome injuries and stayed motivated by following these simple tried-and-true programs. I know you will find yourself on these pages, and no matter your starting point, I'm confident you'll be able to take the steps necessary to do what you want to do, be who you want to be and live your best life.

Happy walking: not only will you be healthier for it, you're going to have fun!

Lynn Kanuka

The following three symbols are used throughout this book:

 Interesting facts about walking, fitness and health

 Brief summaries of key information from the text

 Walking tips from Olympian Lynn Kanuka

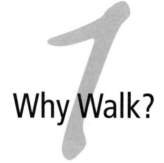

Why Walk?

THE PLAIN AND SIMPLE ANSWER TO THE QUESTION THAT opens this chapter is: the more you move, the healthier you will become and the better you will feel. Walking is, without doubt, one of the easiest ways to improve your health, fitness and overall well-being. For many of us, walking makes up nearly all of our daily activity. And at the end of the day, it's the sum of our steps that determines the state of our health. You may not perceive the few steps to the car or the quick walk home from the grocery store as exercise, but it's the accumulation of this activity, or the lack of it, that can determine whether you're active and healthy or sedentary and unhealthy. From improving your heart health and elevating your mood to maintaining a healthy weight, walking is an ideal form of exercise for almost everyone.

Eleven reasons why walking is great:

1. Anyone can do it.
2. It improves your health.
3. It slows the aging process.
4. It is excellent for heart health.
5. It builds healthy bones.
6. It improves mood and reduces stress.
7. It increases flexibility.
8. It is an effective way to control weight.
9. It is a good form of transportation.
10. It is good for the environment.
11. It is fun and enjoyable.

Anyone Can Do It

If you can put one foot in front of the other, you can walk for exercise. You can do it! Honest. Most people can walk for exercise—whether you've never been active in the past or whether you're recovering from an injury or a health problem. Gradually increasing the number of steps you take each day is a great way to improve your fitness. The best part is that you can do it almost anytime, anywhere, and all you need is a pair of walking shoes and a good dose of motivation to get you on your way.

Walking Improves Your Health

Exercise doesn't have to hurt for it to work. One of the biggest challenges facing individuals who start an exercise program is overcoming the belief that for a fitness routine to be beneficial, it must be rigorous and difficult. The truth is, you just need to become more active than you are currently to begin reaping the rewards. Once you start walking for exercise, you will realize that over time your strength, energy and confidence will improve.

In this book, we provide you with a walking program that is gradual and progressive. Our long-term goal is for you to be able to walk 30 minutes a day, most days of the week. This is the level of activity recommended for general health by the Center for Disease Control and Prevention, the American College of Sports Medicine and the surgeon general of the United States. But don't be concerned if this goal feels out of reach. Remember, this book is a road map for improving your fitness. As with any journey, you get to decide your starting point and your destination.

Every step counts

It might sound almost too good to be true. After all, how can increasing your fitness be as easy as adding extra movement to your day by taking a quick 10-minute walk on your coffee break or by leaving the car at home and walking to work? It is this simple, because every single step counts. The more you move, the fitter and healthier you become. Whether you begin your walking program by taking a jaunt around the block before dinner a couple of nights a week or by taking a 20-minute walk on Sundays with a friend, the point is to get up and get moving—everyone has to start somewhere.

It might not seem like exercise, but it is

Cardiovascular exercise is any continuous rhythmic exercise that uses large muscle groups. This includes

 Be patient
The temptation is always to do too much, too fast and too soon. Walking can be stressful on your body, because there is impact with each step. The body needs time to adjust to the impact of walking. Blasting out the door for your first walk in 4 years isn't the best approach to achieve an improved level of fitness. Instead, you've done the right thing by adopting a well-thought-out, gradual and progressive program. If at first it seems too easy, that's good. You should always feel as if you could have done more.

such activities as walking, jogging, cycling or swimming. A well-exercised heart is able to pump a large amount of blood with fewer beats than a weak heart. A strong heart muscle makes a person more resistant to all sorts of health problems, such as stress and heart attacks. Just as it's good for the heart to be exercised, lack of exercise can be potentially harmful to your health.

Walking Slows the Aging Process

We will all grow old, but research indicates that by maintaining a regular exercise program such as walking, it is possible to prevent as much as 50 percent of the functional decline associated with aging. In other words, this can be the difference between struggling to bend over to tie your shoes and completing a daily 30-minute walk without any aches or pains.

Furthermore, according to the American College of Sports Medicine's *Fit Society* publication, exercise for people 65 years old:

- improves mood and physical well-being
- improves heart and lung function
- decreases the chances of illness
- reduces anxiety and depression
- slows the aging process
- improves muscle strength and endurance
- reduces the risk of osteoporosis
- minimizes the chances of falling

Walking after menopause

Many women are surprised to learn there are significant health benefits to walking after menopause. The

American College of Sports Medicine Web site outlines a recent study that says, "Women 65 or older who increased their physical activity lowered their risk of death during the postmenopausal follow-up period by close to 50 percent." According to this study, for postmenopausal women regular exercise:

- reduces the risk of coronary heart disease by two-thirds
- minimizes bone density loss
- decreases the likelihood of hip fractures associated with falling
- reduces weight gain and minimizes fat accumulation

The benefits for boomers

Baby boomers are the generation of people born between 1946 and 1964. In North America, this is the first generation to understand the connection between being physically active and living a long and healthy life. Boomers, as a group, have been more active than previous generations, but research shows that a large percentage of boomers are overweight and live a sedentary lifestyle.

What are they doing about it? A U.S. study indicates that in 2005 in the United States more than 1.5 million adults aged 55 or older worked with a personal trainer. A separate study shows that adults over 55 are joining health clubs at a higher rate than any other age group. Boomers know that regardless of age, regular exercise has far-reaching benefits, including improved heart health, balance and general attitude about life.

Commitment

Make a personal decision to stick to your program by setting aside the time to walk three times per week, with the longer-term goal of walking for about 30 minutes almost every day. Use your daily planner or your calendar to pencil in your scheduled walking time, the same way you would for any other important appointment. Make exercise a priority just like work and family obligations—it will increase your commitment to your fitness goal.

Ways you can prevent heart disease:

- maintain a healthy weight
- become more active
- reduce high blood pressure
- stop smoking
- lower cholesterol
- limit alcohol
- minimize stress

Health research indicates that people who exercise regularly or have a job that requires them to be constantly on the move suffer fewer heart attacks than people who are significantly less active. As well, those people who are fit and have heart attacks are more likely to survive than their sedentary counterparts.

Walking Is Excellent for Heart Health

It's amazing what a few extra steps a day can do for the health of your heart. Heart disease is among the leading causes of death for men and women. Coronary heart disease is caused by hardening of the arteries, which is a gradual buildup of fatty deposits in the arteries surrounding the heart. These arteries provide the heart with the oxygen and nutrients it requires to pump blood throughout the body. The fatty deposits, over time, can grow and eventually restrict blood flow to the heart muscle. If the blood flow in one or more of the arteries is completely blocked, it can result in heart attack or injury to the heart muscle.

Although heart disease is a serious problem, the good news is that it can be prevented and in some cases reversed. One of the major risk factors for developing heart disease is physical inactivity. According to Health Canada resources, adopting an active lifestyle is the most effective way of reducing the risk of heart disease. As a result, walking more is one of the first steps towards improved heart health. Visit your family physician to discuss your concerns and to make a plan that works for you, especially if you have had a heart attack or angina or if tests have revealed that you have clogged arteries.

Walking Builds Healthy Bones

As we age, our bones have a tendency to become weak and fragile. Women especially are at risk of developing osteoporosis, a condition that is characterized by a decrease in bone mass and bone density and increases the susceptibility to painful bone fractures.

Osteoporosis often has psychological and social consequences, such as depression, fear of falling and social withdrawal.

According to Dr. Teresa Liu-Ambrose, assistant professor at the University of British Columbia and a member of the UBC Bone Health Research Group, exercise has a role in promoting healthy bones across a person's life span. Bone health is affected by genetics, estrogen and other systemic hormones, age, gender, diet, lifestyle factors, medications and physical activity. For example, certain lifestyle factors, such as smoking, and consuming caffeine and alcohol, are associated with high calcium losses. Alcohol abuse is a strong risk factor associated with bone loss. To minimize the risk of low bone density or to increase your existing bone density, most forms of exercise are found to be a strong influence on bone strength and mass. Dr. Liu-Ambrose notes that participating in a regular walking program, such as the ones in this book, has been proven to be effective in improving bone mass density of the spine and the hip.

Walking Improves Mood and Reduces Stress

Walking is good for the heart and soul. Taking a break from work to go outside for a breath of fresh air and a walk around the block is an effective way to clear your head from the stresses of life. Walking, or any form of exercise, definitely helps to elevate mood and decrease stress, which is why physicians often recommend regular exercise as a way to keep the blues away as well as to combat minor bouts of depression. During exercise the

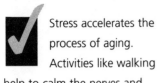

Stress accelerates the process of aging. Activities like walking help to calm the nerves and alleviate tension.

brain releases endorphins, which are brain chemicals that can stimulate relaxation. Basically, endorphins help you to achieve naturally what many antidepressant medications do artificially. Walking, even at a slow pace, can trigger the release of endorphins and in turn make you happier and more relaxed.

It's likely that you've experienced some form of stress such as irregular sleep patterns, lack of appetite, irritability, anxiety and general tension. Walking (or any cardiovascular exercise) is an effective way to relax your nerves and reduce your stress levels. Even if it's just for a short period of time, regular walks can provide an escape from mental stress. Exercising during stressful periods gives you the opportunity to process thoughts and release negativity. This combination of thought processing and endorphins often allows you to create an optimistic outlook, which keeps you from feeling anxious or depressed. A positive attitude can also improve your immune system. When you do anything physical, even a short walk around the block, it refreshes you and gives you an energy boost. It is also a reminder that you are alive!

Walking Increases Flexibility

One of the most common reasons for not exercising is the fear of tripping and falling that might lead to an injury. As we age, our bones lose strength and mass, and our soft tissues—our muscles, tendons and ligaments—become less elastic and more prone to tearing. Stretching is a great way to loosen up your muscles. According to Louisiana sport medicine physician

Walking for Fitness

Dr. Bryan Barootes, "Seniors who have been previously sedentary are often faced with balance and strength problems." He strongly believes that a gradual walking program helps to improve strength and balance, and by regularly stretching your main muscle areas you will improve your flexibility—the ability of muscles and joints to move through their full range of motion.

If you include stretching exercises in your fitness program, your muscles will become more pliable and decrease your chances of injury. The more flexible you are, the better your balance and the less likely you will be to trip and fall. As well, good flexibility adds to your overall enjoyment in walking and performing regular

 If you're an aging senior who wants to increase your flexibility, hold on to a railing or another stable support and try balancing on one foot while waiting in the grocery store lineup, or try rising up on your toes several times—every different or extra movement like these throughout the course of your day will move your body towards greater flexibility, strength and improved fitness.

WALKER PROFILE

Dan

Dan is a 42-year-old office administrator who has had great success in taking the slow and steady approach to weight management. About 2 years ago he realized that he weighed over 200 pounds (91 kilograms), which was significantly heavier than what he saw as a healthy weight for his small frame. After speaking with a few friends who are physicians, Dan realized that if he didn't make changes to his lifestyle and eating habits, he would continue his walk towards obesity. These same friends also warned him about the far-reaching health concerns associated with obesity, such as diabetes and heart disease. Dan says, "My parents are in their sixties and they don't have any health problems. I didn't want to be another obesity statistic. Also, I hated the feeling of being overweight."

Once Dan realized that he needed to lose some weight, he spoke with his wife about changing his diet, and she was immediately supportive. Dan made the decision to eat smaller portions and to make an effort to get a greater balance of protein, carbohydrates, fruits and vegetables. He now walks for exercise four to five times a week for 30 minutes. During the week, most of Dan's exercise is done during his lunch break at a local health club, where he walks on the treadmill. On the weekends, he does his banking and grocery shopping on foot, as he finds this to be an easy way to get in some exercise while taking care of his errands. Dan says, "Weight loss isn't a secret. It's about regular exercise and eating a balanced diet."

Thin isn't always in. Keep in mind that thin doesn't necessarily mean healthy. After all, we all know of thin people who smoke, eat poorly and drink an excessive amount of alcohol. Instead, if you focus on your behavior and make relatively small changes to your activity level, you can have a significant positive impact on your health risks.

daily activities such as going up stairs and gardening. In addition to using the walking program in this book, it's a good idea to regularly include a thorough stretching routine at the end of your walk. For suggestions on a proper stretching routine, refer to appendix A.

Walking Is an Effective Way to Control Weight

Yes! Walking will help you manage your weight. If you are interested in making some changes to your weight, it's important to first understand that weight gain occurs when you take in more calories than you expend. For example, if you regularly take in 100 calories more a day than you expend, this means a weight gain of roughly 10 pounds (4.5 kilograms) per year. Restricting your food intake may lead to short-term weight loss but on its own it is not a long-term solution. As an active person who walks, you need food to maintain your energy and your desire to exercise.

Sandy Friedman, a counselor and writer in the field of eating disorder and prevention, believes people focus too much attention on their weight. "Focusing only on what the scale tells you can be detrimental to people's self-esteem and long-term success. Too often self-esteem is tied to an arbitrary number, which can result in people feeling as though 'I'm not good enough as I am,'" says Friedman. Instead, she encourages people to focus on feeling strong instead of on weight loss. In other words, by saying to yourself "I want to become healthier and fitter" instead of "I want to weigh 145 pounds (66 kilograms)," you are more likely to experience

Walking for Fitness

feelings of success and to feel good about yourself and your body. Everyone's genetic history is individual, which means that maintaining a healthy body weight is as different and unique as the person. Your genetic profile, sociocultural upbringing and socioeconomic status are factors in determining your body shape and size. For information and suggestions on walking for weight control, turn to chapter 5.

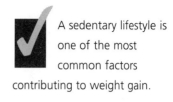 A sedentary lifestyle is one of the most common factors contributing to weight gain.

Walking Is a Good Form of Transportation

Use your feet to commute. By using your feet instead of the car, you can make mundane tasks and errands a lot more enjoyable. In an ideal world you will be able to easily set aside 30 minutes to walk, five to six times a week, but many of you might not have this sort of luxury or

WALKER PROFILE

Mary

Mary, a retired nurse and special-needs instructor, is far from your average 75-year-old. On most days, she walks for about 60 minutes along her favorite path, overlooking the Pacific Ocean. Walking alone is Mary's preference, as she enjoys the solitude and the freedom of dictating her own pace.

Originally from Britain, Mary often walked as a means of transportation when her children were younger since the family had one car, which was used for her husband's work. When she moved to Canada, Mary continued to stay active with regular walking and cycling.

Ten years ago, Mary was diagnosed with bladder cancer. Many people in a similar situation would have stopped exercising, but Mary walked for pleasure throughout most of her cancer treatment. A few years later, at age 69, she was faced with breast cancer. With the support and love of her husband and family, she endured a lumpectomy, radiation and chemotherapy. Again, she continued walking. Mary says, "I love the outdoors, and I was happy to have my husband join me for many of my walks during that time. I just feel so fortunate to have walking as a hobby, to be given the gift of living in the pristine environment of the Pacific Northwest."

Mary's positive attitude, passion for walking and no-excuses attitude is definitely a motivation for anyone interested in improving their health and fitness!

flexibility in your work or family responsibilities. With a little creative planning, you can easily add more steps to each day. Here are a few simple suggestions for using your feet more and your car less:

- If you need to pick up some milk at the corner store or you want to rent a DVD for the weekend, leave your car at home and use your feet.
- On the weekends, plan to meet friends for lunch or brunch at a restaurant that is within walking distance of your house. If you will work up a sweat on your walk to the restaurant, take a change of clothes in your backpack to put on when you arrive. You can walk home after your meal or plan to have one of your friends drive you home.
- If you have a passion for gardening, find some homes with inspiring gardens and take a walk along the street so you can get some ideas that you can incorporate into your own garden.
- One of your hobbies might be looking at houses in beautiful or unique neighborhoods. If you see a street that interests you, stop and take a walk or make the street part of a new walking route.

Walking Is Good for the Environment

Using your feet as a means of commuting is not only good for your health, it's also great for the health of the environment. According to award-winning scientist, environmentalist and broadcaster Dr. David Suzuki, "Sustainability means living within the earth's limits. Living in a world where feeding the people does not necessitate polluting groundwater and coastal shorelines. Where transporting people and goods does not mean polluting the air and changing the climate."

Living in a sustainable way means taking more responsibility for the choices you make and how you live. This includes everything from what you eat and where you live to the relationship you have with nature. What does sustainability have to do with walking? Plenty. By making a commitment to drive less and walk more, you are effectively improving not only your health but also the air you breathe. It's estimated that about 50 percent of car use is for trips within 3 miles (5 kilometers) of home. For many of you, this is within walking range.

i Replacing short car trips with walking is an easy way to get in the recommended 30 minutes of physical activity you need each day for good health and weight management. Remember, your half hour of exercise can be an accumulation of three 10-minute walks; this might be an easier and more effective way to get in your exercise.

Walking Is Fun and Enjoyable

Most people who walk regularly have made it an enjoyable part of their lifestyle. Some people may find walking with friends and family members to be a great way to stay connected while getting some exercise. Others may find they want the solace and peace of mind that often accompanies walking alone. Regardless of whether walking is for solitude or socialization, the point is to make it enjoyable for you.

Make walking fun

Here are some suggestions for making walking more fun:

- If you like the outdoors and love being with nature, find a green space, park or trail near your home and enjoy a short walk in this environment. Most communities offer one of these settings.
- Socializing with friends might be what you're looking

for, in which case you could ask a friend or family member to meet you. After a couple of walks together, you might consider organizing a regular time when the two of you could meet up for your walk.

- If you live in an area with extremely hot weather conditions, consider walking in the early morning hours to avoid the midday heat. Or, if you're in a cold-weather climate, try walking in shopping malls or on a treadmill at your local community center.

- Get to know your community. City streets with trees, well-maintained sidewalks and proper lighting are

Kenji

Kenji is a 49-year-old events coordinator with the San Francisco gay and lesbian society. Recently, he was asked to organize a walking group for bereaved widows. He had never heard of walking groups, let alone specifically for widows. Kenji researched walking groups online and was surprised to learn that they are in huge demand. When he posted a sign on the bulletin board at work and sent a brief e-mail to society members, he was overwhelmed by the interest in his own new 9-week walking program.

Kenji's research suggested that he should have several trained volunteers accompany the walking group. There would be one volunteer for every three walkers, and it would be the role of the volunteers to ensure that participants never walked alone. A few weeks before the program start date, Kenji organized a volunteer-training session with a bereavement counselor. All of the volunteers had lost a friend or family member, so they were ideal volunteer walk leaders.

On the first Sunday of the program, the participants met at a beautiful park in the city. Each week thereafter they assembled at a different greenway in order to keep the walks interesting and to explore various neighborhoods. Most of the participants attended the entire 9-week program, finding the group a great opportunity to be with others who were experiencing a similar loss. The program was such a success that at the end of the 9 weeks, the group decided to continue its weekly walks. Since that first group, Kenji has received so many requests for both bereavement and regular walking groups that he now runs five groups a year.

Walking for Fitness

good places for walking. Neighborhood stores, restaurants and banks are easily accessible on foot. Many of these communities also offer a variety of places to walk, such as dirt and grass trails, greenways, and schools or colleges with outdoor tracks.

- If you live in an urban center surrounded by more concrete and cars than trees and green grass, consider driving or taking public transit to a neighborhood that is more enjoyable for walking.

Walk to the latest hits

If you dislike walking on busy streets crowded with cars and people, you might try using a headset or an iPod to listen to your favorite songs. Music can make your walks more enjoyable, and you're less likely to focus on surrounding noise. A word of caution: if you do decide to use a headset, it's important to keep your safety in mind. You need to be aware of your surroundings at all times. For this reason, walking at night while wearing a headset is not the safest idea, but enjoying your favorite hits while commuting on foot to work should be okay during daylight hours when the streets are busy with other pedestrians. Another idea for music lovers is to walk on a treadmill at the local gym—it's a great way to get fit and enjoy your tunes while staying out of harm's way.

 Top Ten Walking Tunes

1. "The Walk"—The Cure
2. "Walk of Life"—Dire Straits
3. "Walk the Line"—Johnny Cash
4. "Walkin' in the Sunshine"—Roger Miller or Frank Sinatra
5. "Walk Tall"—John Mellencamp
6. "Walking Man"—James Taylor
7. "Walk On"—U2
8. "These Boots Are Made for Walkin'"—Nancy Sinatra
9. "I Want to Walk You Home"—Fats Domino
10. "Walk"—Burning Spear

Getting Started

IT'S TIME TO PUT YOUR BEST FOOT FORWARD. HUFFING and puffing doesn't have to describe your fitness program. You probably don't have to look far to see walkers of every size and age imaginable, moving along at various speeds while enjoying the beauty of the outdoors. These fit folks aren't gasping for breath as they make their way along the trail or sidewalk; rather, they are relaxed and invigorated. But don't fool yourself into thinking that an active lifestyle is easy and effortless for everyone except you. Even high-level athletes have days or weeks where they struggle to get out the door for their run or their bike ride. With a solid walking plan, an understanding of some of the common roadblocks to maintaining a regular walking program and a commitment to keep at it... you will be well on your way to improved health and fitness.

Visit Your Doctor

Your health and safety should be your most important priority. A regular walking program can build almost anyone's fitness foundation as long as you take the proper precautions. Dr. Bryan Barootes, a sport medicine physician, encourages anyone embarking on a

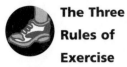

The Three Rules of Exercise

1. Moderation: Be patient and resist doing too much too soon. Find a program that starts at the right level for you and increases your walking distance very gradually so you can avoid injury.

2. Consistency: Use a set schedule such as the walking program outlined in this book. It may sound rigid, but you are more likely to stay on track and meet your goals in a safe and gradual manner.

3. Rest: Give your body time to recover. Exercise puts stress on the body, so it's a good idea when you're first starting out to allow for at least one rest day between the days you walk.

new fitness program to first visit their family doctor. "A thorough health review and physical exam to screen for medical problems or to identify limitations or restrictions of chronic medical problems is a must for previously sedentary people. Individuals with known chronic problems such as diabetes, emphysema, heart disease and vascular disease should definitely have an assessment by their family physician and be advised regarding the intensity of their exercise program. Your physician may require some blood tests or other investigations depending on results of the screening or medical problems," says Dr. Barootes. The Physical Activity Readiness Questionnaire (PAR-Q) in appendix B is an excellent screening tool, but he recommends that anyone over the age of 50 undergo a thorough medical exam.

Rule 1: Moderation

Slow down. Walking is one of the easiest activities in terms of convenience, but jumping into an intensive walking program after being sedentary for months or even years is simply not safe. "It's my experience that most people tend to push themselves too hard," says Dr. Barootes. "When you begin a walking program, for the most part you should always be able to carry on a conversation with a friend." For long-term success, it's important to gradually increase your walking distance and speed.

Rule 2: Consistency

To get the most out of your walking program and to gain the greatest health benefits, you need to be consis-

Walking for Fitness

tent. Walking is like anything in life—whether it's school, career or learning a new sport, consistency is the key to success. By maintaining a consistent walking program like the ones outlined in this book, you are able to safely and gradually change your fitness habits and lifestyle patterns. The idea is that over time these new patterns will become second nature, and you'll be well on your way to an active lifestyle.

Rule 3: Rest

You need time to rest and recover from your walks in order to get fitter, stronger and healthier. It takes time for your muscles, bones and ligaments to adjust to the impact of a consistent walking schedule, so you will need to listen to your body and respond accordingly. If you still feel sore on a scheduled walk day, take an extra day off and delay your walk session for the following day. This helps to avoid burnout and overuse injuries (see chapter 6).

Commonly Asked Questions from Beginning Walkers

Q. *How far should I walk my first time out?*

A. The answer to this question depends on your level of fitness. Some people have never maintained a regular walking program but they regularly garden, play golf and shovel snow from the walk. Others carry a significant amount of body fat and have difficulty walking from the house to the car and back again. Your first step is to speak with your health care provider about your walking goals. Together you can assess your level of fitness, then review the guidelines in this chapter and

***i* Use your arms**

With regular walking, you will gradually find a comfortable rhythm, and your technique will improve as you become stronger. Working on core strength will help as well. Generally, try to walk tall, keep your shoulders square, hold your stomach muscles strong, maintain a strong heel-toe motion and focus on moving forward. Also, don't forget to use your arms: they dictate your pace and rhythm and will keep you going. If you consciously think about pumping your arms, your legs will follow.

the walking program in chapter 3 and determine your own starting point.

Q. *Should I walk every day?*

A. No. If you are new to walking for fitness, you will want to avoid walking on consecutive days, especially at the beginning. Having a rest day between a workout or walk day gives your body and mind time to recover. Eventually, walking will become easier, and you may reach a point where you can walk on back-to-back days, but for many of you, regular physical activity is a new challenge.

Q. *What will walking for exercise feel like?*

A. If you are starting an exercise program after being inactive for an extended period of time, you're bound to experience some initial fatigue, stiffness and possibly soreness. However, if you follow the gradual program outlined in this book, you will progress at a slow but careful rate that reduces your chances of fatigue, injury and boredom. Keep in mind that your goal is to improve your health and fitness by creating a walking lifestyle that you can enjoy and maintain in the long term.

Choosing a Walking Program

It might seem silly or rigid to set out a walking program for yourself. After all, can't you just tie up your old sneakers and head out the door? Of course you can, but whether you're an elite athlete or someone getting off the couch for the first time in years, you need to create a fitness plan that will work for you. Once your physician

Walking for Fitness

confirms that you can proceed with a walking program, you want to start with what's comfortable for you. Everyone's fitness level is different, so it's important not to get caught up in comparing yourself with anyone else. How far and how fast should you walk? This book is designed to help you set goals and create a structured walking plan to get you going and to stay walking well into the future.

Knowing where to start

The walking program outlined in the next chapter is gradual and progressive, which allows you to start at a point in the program that matches your current fitness level. For example, a person who occasionally walks for

Brady

Brady is a 25-year-old stockbroker who lost over 50 pounds (23 kilograms) after he started dating a woman he met through an online relationship service. After seeing Brandee's picture and reading about her interests, hobbies and career aspirations, he sent her the first of many e-mails. Brady had not been on a date in almost 3 years, and the long hours at work, excessive amounts of late-night takeout food and little exercise made him self-conscious, especially at the thought of dating someone as fit and attractive as Brandee. But, after a few weeks of online chatting, they agreed to meet in person and immediately connected.

Brandee was clearly fitter than Brady, but her positive attitude encouraged Brady to join a health club with the goal of getting fit and losing weight. Initially, he tried to get to the gym every night after work and walk for 20 minutes on the treadmill before doing some stationary weight training. But after 2 weeks he was exhausted and frustrated about not losing any weight.

After Brady skipped a few days of exercise, Brandee gently raised the topic of trying to do too much too soon and encouraged him to forget about losing weight and instead focus on moving more. Brady thought about her suggestions and revised his goals: he made getting to the gym three times a week his short-term goal and walked to work on the days he didn't go to the gym. These days Brady is happier with his weight but, more than anything, he likes the feeling of being fit and doing active things with Brandee.

i Having a good sport watch is helpful. Most sport watches are lightweight, weatherproof, easy to see and have various features to easily keep track of the time you spend walking.

about half an hour on weekends would start the walking program at the beginning. If you walk more regularly, you would start at a point farther into the program.

Starting from scratch

Maybe you've been sedentary for a long time and you're not quite ready to start the walking program in chapter 3—that's okay. Remember, the point isn't where you start, but that you have the courage to take the first step. If this describes your current fitness level, you might be tempted to create your own program. This is fine, but it's still a good idea to use some general guidelines that will support you on your journey towards a more active lifestyle. Dr. Bryan Barootes is a big proponent of walking for fitness, health and lifestyle, and he's developed the following slow and gradual approach for those who have been sedentary for an extended period and are working towards a walking program (see also chapter 3, Phase 1: First Steps):

• Start by walking 5 to 10 minutes every other day for 1 to 2 weeks. Walk wherever is comfortable and convenient—in your house, on a treadmill, at a mall or outside. Walk at the pace of a "southern amble," which means a gentle, leisurely stroll.

• If you haven't encountered any problems, increase your walking time by 3 to 5 minutes every 2 to 3 weeks.

• Once you can walk continuously for 20 minutes at a time, you can begin phase 3 of the walking program in chapter 3 or continue with Dr. Barootes' general guidelines and add an additional day to your weekly walk schedule every 3 to 4 weeks until you are walking 5 days a week. Increase your pace to a "brisk military walk."

• Once you are able to walk for 20 minutes, 5 days a week, increase the duration of your walk to 30 minutes a day.

• Take the "start low and go slow" approach and you will be more likely to achieve your exercise goals.

When to Walk

The first step in any exercise program, after getting the okay to exercise from your family doctor, is to create a plan that will work for you. A good plan—one that builds your fitness gradually and fits with your current lifestyle—will help you meet your goal. It doesn't matter when or even where you walk; you just need to create and maintain a consistent walking routine that easily fits into your daily life. After answering some of the following questions, you should be able to formulate your own personal walking plan:

- Are you an early riser or a night owl? If you have difficulty getting out of bed before 8:00 AM, an early morning walking program might not be the best idea for you. Instead, consider other options such as walking during your lunch break, walking home from work or walking after dinner with the dog.

- What are some of the other demands on your time? Try to figure out what time during the week and on weekends you can use for walking. Be realistic and creative in making time to walk. Consider walking to work one way and taking the bus home. Commuting on foot is an efficient way to stay committed to your walking goals.

- Do you enjoy visiting with friends and family? If so, you could make walking part of your get-togethers or ask a friend or family member to join you for one of your walks. Or, if you don't have anyone in your life who wants to walk with you, ask about walking groups at your community center or local health club.

Find a walking friend

You need support. It can be motivating and fun to do your walking workout with a friend, a group or a canine. But make sure that your friend likes to move at about the same pace as you do.

Ten ways to work walking into your day:

1. Take the stairs instead of the elevator.
2. Walk your child to school or to play dates.
3. Do your errands on foot instead of taking the car. Walk to your dentist appointment and as many other appointments as possible.
4. Walk to a local restaurant for lunch with your friends, and walk home afterward.
5. Walk home from work. Or stroll in the park during spring and summer months and walk in the mall during the colder days of winter and fall.
6. After dinner, instead of watching TV, walk to a friend's house and back—each way could be 10 minutes, which would give you 20 minutes of walking.
7. Offer to walk a friend's dog, or volunteer to exercise the dogs at your local pet shelter.
8. Join a bird-watching group. It's likely that there will be at least some walking involved. It's a great way to get outside, meet new people and get some exercise while learning about birds.
9. Choose fun activities that require energy, such as dancing or bicycling.
10. If you must drive, park farther away than you need to so that you force yourself to walk the extra distance.

Where to Walk

Most of us have numerous choices of where we can walk—in our neighborhood, around a local park, on a treadmill or inside a shopping mall. Where you walk is not as important as finding places that will meet your needs, interests and current fitness level.

Indoors versus outdoors

Take some time to plan where you will do your initial few walks, so it's one less thing you have to think about when you head out the door. Whether you walk indoors or outdoors, both are great ways to get fit and improve your health. Keep in mind that even if you plan to walk outside most of the time, you can always start your walking program inside, build your strength, fitness and confidence, and then move outdoors once you're ready. Or you can walk inside when it's too hot, cold or rainy or if it's too late in the day to walk safely outside.

Mall walking

At first glance, mall walking may seem a little silly or boring. But malls don't have hills or too many stairs, which minimizes your chances of tripping and falling. Also, there are washrooms, places to sit and rest, and the mall security provides a safe environment. An added bonus is that you can easily reward yourself with a post-walk coffee or tea from one of the food court vendors. Make mall walking more interesting by inviting along a friend to chat with. Or make a point of going when the stores are open, so you can do some window shopping. It's likely that you will see at least a couple of people walking for exercise. Ask whether your mall provides incentives such as health checkups, discounts and mileage rewards for walkers and walking groups.

Vary the places you choose to walk

Be creative! If you want to avoid boredom, keep your walks interesting by including variety. Find the quiet streets, beautiful parks and soft trails in your neighborhood. Walking on hilly trails or up stairs will definitely increase the challenge and intensity of your walks, and varied terrain can prevent injury as you alter the angles at which your limbs absorb impact. For suggestions on good places to walk, ask at the fitness store where you purchase walking shoes and clothing.

Treadmills

If you've heard yourself saying that you're too busy with work and family demands to exercise regularly, treadmill walking might be the answer. Treadmill walking is basically walking in one place. As a result, treadmills are easy to use, provide great flexibility so you can exercise when you want, stay dry and warm and even catch up on the television news or watch a movie. You also get the same aerobic benefits as from regular walking. In fact, according to a study published in the *Journal of the American Medical Association,* "treadmills easily outpace an exercise bicycle, a rowing machine and a cross-country ski machine." Most treadmill models add consistency to your exercise routine by allowing you to maintain a specific speed and intensity throughout your workout. Also, most machines keep track of the time and distance, making it simple to monitor the duration of your walks as well as your overall progress.

Many gyms and community centers have treadmills you can use, but if you're really short on time and are committed to your walking program, you can also buy your own. Being able to exercise with your child in close range is time efficient and adds flexibility to your family's schedule. How else could you supermoms and -dads do a load of laundry, bake a cake, watch your child and walk for 30 minutes all at the same time! And, if you have safety or health concerns that make it difficult for you to exercise regularly outside or at a gym, this might be one way to stay active within the safety of your own home.

Indoor tracks

Many universities, large recreation centers and private gyms have indoor tracks. These facilities will likely charge a user's fee, but they're a safe way to walk at night and avoid hills and stairs as well as the smog and traffic of city streets. Unlike treadmills, indoor tracks allow you to walk alongside a walking partner, so you can easily socialize while completing your workout.

Neighborhoods

Walking in your neighborhood can be a great way to get to know who lives there and what's going on. It's also a practical way to build your walking program gradually.

Karl

Karl is a computer programmer who turned 55 last year. In the lead-up to his birthday, he started going to his local YMCA. He's an outgoing guy with some good friends, but he joined a gym to get fit, lose a little weight and meet others who live in his community.

After a few months, Karl was starting to feel fitter, and he was intrigued by the number of people he had met who shared similar goals of fitness and weight loss. What he found surprising was how few of them maintained a regular exercise program for more than a month or so. He says, "In speaking with others at my gym, I came to understand that when people first start an exercise program, they often make the mistake of thinking that they will, in the first week or two, begin to lose their desired weight. When they don't, most of the folks I've met become frustrated and often give up." Karl believes that many of them have unrealistic expectations.

It took Karl a few months of consistent walking and weight training 4 days a week before he started to lose weight. He too was initially frustrated by how long it took his body to respond to his fitness routine, but he did notice a difference in his energy level and welcomed the change from working in front of a computer all day. These days Karl realizes that he needs to maintain a routine to stay on track: if he doesn't have time to go to the gym, he usually walks around his neighborhood for 20 to 30 minutes.

Create a walking route on quiet streets that circles past your house. That way, if your goal is to walk for 30 minutes, you can fashion a 10-minute loop and do it three times. If you decide after two loops that you've had enough, you're close to home and you won't have to worry about being stranded. After a while your fitness will improve and so will your confidence. For obvious safety reasons, always tell someone where you're walking and when you'll be home. Carry your cell phone or change for the pay phone in the event that you need to call a cab.

To make your outdoor walks safer and more enjoyable, look for neighborhoods with good sidewalks. If you're just starting out, try to avoid hills and stairs that can cause you to twist or strain your ankles and knees. Walk during the daylight hours, or when walking at night or in the early morning hours take a friend, carry a flashlight or headlamp or stick to well-lit paths.

In the winter months, try to walk on shoveled streets. Ice and snow can be slippery, so you want to be extra careful not to trip and fall. If you're going to be doing a significant amount of winter walking, it might be a good idea to invest in a second pair of walking shoes. Ask the knowledgeable salesperson at your local athletic-shoe store for suggestions—trail runners have good treads and might help you to maneuver along the snowy streets.

Outdoor tracks

Try walking on the outdoor track at your local high school. These are usually soft and smooth, which will minimize your chances of falling. Be sure to use the outside lane, and watch for runners and speed walkers.

Tips for Walking Safety

There are two dangers to consider when walking on city streets: motorists and predators (human and animal!). With some careful planning you can minimize both dangers.

- Wear bright-colored clothing—white is best!—so you're visible to motorists even in low light or poor weather.

- Buy outerwear with reflective stripes and patches that are noticeable enough that a passing car can quickly see you.

- Purchase small lights that attach to your waist, leg or arm. Most running or cycling stores offer low-cost lights that are lightweight and made for this purpose.

- Carry a handheld flashlight to make yourself noticeable and to more easily spot dips in the road. Headlamps like the ones worn by underground miners are also great for night walking, because they are bright and allow you to move your hands freely.

- Make eye contact with the car drivers at a crosswalk or driveway before crossing. Don't ever trust that every driver will look before turning right, especially at a red light.

- Walk on sidewalks rather than on the road during the evening or early morning hours. Always walk facing traffic, so that you can see the approaching headlights and, if need be, move off the road.

Set yourself up to succeed

There's no secret pill or shortcut to becoming fit, but if you incorporate the three keys to any successful exercise program—moderation, consistency and rest—you're guaranteed to be successful. It may not happen immediately, but, if you are patient and remember the three rules, over time your daily walks will become a pleasure rather than an obligation riddled with difficulty and dread.

- Avoid dark alleys, poorly lit streets and unpopular areas of the city, especially when walking at night. Trust your intuition if you feel unsafe or if someone seems suspicious at any time.
- Ask a friend or family member to join you for your evening walk or take the dog with you, as there is safety in numbers, especially for women.
- Vary your walking routes as well as the time of day you walk, so that criminals cannot easily predict your routine and plan an attack.
- Carry a cell phone, change for the pay phone and identification, so that you can contact the police or someone you trust in case of emergency.
- Take precautions such as keeping the volume low if

Judy

Judy is a retired nurse who has been an avid golfer for almost 50 years. Over the years she's used walking as a way to stay fit for the hilly 18-hole golf course she plays almost daily during the spring and summer months. When asked how she's stayed motivated to maintain a high level of fitness, Judy says, "I've found walking to have so many benefits. The social, psychological and health benefits are motivators for me to continue with a regular routine. Walking also puts me in a good mood, and it's been a great way to maintain my weight."

About 10 years ago, Judy had a walking partner who encouraged her to join a hiking group. At first she hesitated, but after one hike with the group she was hooked. In the past several years she has tackled some challenging local hikes in the Selkirk and Rocky mountain ranges that surround the small mining community she calls home. In order to build stamina and strength for hiking, Judy maintains a regular weight-training program in addition to walking three to four times a week. Most of her walks take her about 40 minutes to complete, with the exception of a 60-minute route she walks once a week. Now that she's approaching her late sixties, she's surprised at the level of activity she continues to maintain. Walking has definitely slowed down the aging process for her, and she's more inspired than ever to continue exploring the great mountain ranges of British Columbia.

Walking for Fitness

you want to listen to music, so that you can remain alert to what's going on in your surroundings.

Choosing a Good Shoe

There are many different types of walking shoes on the market today. According to Phil Moore, a sport-shoe specialist in Vancouver, B.C., "Many of the shoes you see today that are marketed as walking shoes are for folks who are destination walkers. Basically they are people who want comfort but need a shoe that also matches their casual or work clothes." For some of you, fashion and style are factors in deciding your footwear, but when it comes to walking for exercise, a good shoe can mean the difference between comfort and pain. You want to be sure to purchase a shoe that will work for you.

Walking versus running shoes

The walking gait differs from the running motion in one very distinct way. When you're walking, one foot is always on the ground, whereas when running, you are airborne for a split second between the time one foot lands and the other one pushes off. As a result, your heel strikes the ground with the force of one to two times your bodyweight when you're walking, compared with three to five times your body weight when you're running. Because of this difference, running shoes generally offer more cushioning and support than the average walking-shoe model. For tips on purchasing your walking shoes, refer to appendix C.

Choosing Your Clothing

Shoes are the only essential item of clothing needed to begin walking, but you will want to dress comfortably. Most of you will have a T-shirt, a sweatshirt and a pair of comfortable pants that you can wear for your first few walks. If you find that you're happy with your current wardrobe, then stick with it. If you find that you do need to buy a few articles of clothing in order to be comfortable on your walks, it's a good idea to spend a little time at your local athletic-clothing store. Many walkers like loose-fitting shirts and pants (or capris) that are lightweight and breathable. Look for synthetic materials that dry quickly and don't chafe, and don't forget to think about your socks and underwear, too. For warmer and cooler days, you may want a cap and a lightweight jacket. Most exercise stores should have a variety of options for you.

If you plan to walk at night, look for clothing in visible colors (white is best) with lots of reflectors so that cars can spot you. If fashion isn't your number 1 concern, consider a low-cost vest, similar to the ones worn by school crosswalk guards or construction workers. Most large department stores or hardware stores will have something suitable. For more detailed information on the benefits of walking-specific clothing, see chapter 6.

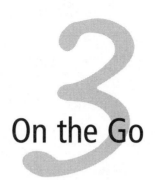

On the Go

READY, SET, GO. NO MATTER HOW MUCH OR HOW LITTLE you exercise, there are universal principles for fitness that form the structure of every good training program. Fitness is like everything else in life: if you use the right building blocks, it almost guarantees a sound structure that will last in the years to come. From warming up to cooling down and everything in between, this chapter provides you with a framework for getting fit and meeting your walking goals. All you need to do is lace up your shoes and head out the door.

Why Walking Programs Work

The walking program in this chapter will form the framework for you to begin walking your way to improved fitness, health and lifestyle. Using a walking program instead of a haphazard approach helps you to establish a walking plan, a detailed schedule as to when, where and how far you will walk. Remember that improved health and fitness require discipline, consistency and commitment. For the most part, the walkers you see on your city streets are just like everyone else—they are fit and healthy because they made a commitment and stuck to it. You may not believe it now, but after completing each session, you will see that you are one step closer to achieving your walking goal. As well, you will see that over time your confidence will increase and you'll find each successful walk session provides positive reinforcement that you too can walk alongside the fitness enthusiasts in your community.

The lifestyle walking program in this chapter consists of four phases. Each phase starts slowly, and during the first few weeks you may find it overly easy. Don't be tempted to skip ahead: even the most experienced walkers need to take a gradual approach to increasing their fitness levels. Doing too much too soon may result in injury and prevent you from continuing the program and ultimately achieving your goal. The program encourages consistency, which allows the body to adjust gradually to a higher fitness level. When you walk regularly from one week to the next, your body has more time to adapt to the stress of training and in turn become stronger and more efficient. If you miss too many training days, your endurance will decrease and your likelihood of injury will increase.

Once you have selected the walking program that's right for you, you might want to make a photocopy to post on your fridge at home or on your bulletin board at work.

Let's Get Started: Lifestyle Walking Program

Phase 1: First Steps

Is this YOU? "I have been completely inactive for an extended period of time." If not, perhaps phase 2 describes your current activity level.

Goal: To take the first steps to a healthier, active lifestyle by working towards walking up to 10 minutes every other day.

	CHALLENGE	DAY 1	DAY 2	DAY 3	DAY 4	DAY 5	DAY 6	DAY 7
WK 1	Off the couch	Walk 5 min.	REST	Walk 5 min.	REST	Walk 7 min.	REST	REST
WK 2	Out the door	Walk 5 min.	REST	Walk 7 min.	REST	Walk 10 min.	REST	REST
WK 3	Around the block	Walk 10 min.	REST	Walk 5 min.	REST	Walk 10 min.	REST	REST
WK 4	Recovery	Walk 5 min.	REST	Walk 10 min.	REST	Walk 7 min.	REST	REST
WK 5	Are you ready for more?	Walk 10 min.	REST	Walk 10 min.	REST	Walk 10 min.	REST	REST

"Am I ready to move to the next phase?" If you don't encounter any difficulties, you're ready for phase 2. If you're not comfortable, repeat the 5-week phase 1 program until you can comfortably walk 10 minutes every other day.

Phase 2: Make a Start

Is this YOU? "I've successfully worked through phase 1." Or "I am generally inactive, but I do go for a short walk around the block once in a while without any difficulties." If you are more active than this, have a look at phase 3.

Goal: To continue with or make a good start on a healthy, active lifestyle by working towards walking for 20 minutes, 5 days a week.

	CHALLENGE	DAY 1	DAY 2	DAY 3	DAY 4	DAY 5	DAY 6	DAY 7
WK 1	Make a start	Walk 10 min.	REST	Walk 15 min.	REST	Walk 10 min.	REST	REST
WK 2	Keep it going	Walk 15 min.	Walk 10 min.	Walk 10 min.	REST	Walk 15 min.	REST	REST
WK 3	Starting to work	Walk 10 min.	Walk 10 min.	Walk 15 min.	REST	Walk 20 min.	REST	REST
WK 4	Recovery	Walk 10 min.	Walk 10 min.	Walk 15 min.	REST	Walk 10 min.	REST	REST
WK 5	Back to work	Walk 10 min.	Walk 10 min.	Walk 15 min.	REST	Walk 20 min.	Walk 10 min.	REST
WK 6	Finding my rhythm	Walk 15 min.	Walk 15 min.	Walk 20 min.	REST	Walk 20 min.	Walk 15 min.	REST
WK 7	Pushing myself a little	Walk 20 min.	Walk 15 min.	Walk 20 min.	REST	Walk 20 min.	Walk 15 min.	REST
WK 8	I can do this!	Walk 20 min.	Walk 20 min.	Walk 20 min.	REST	Walk 20 min.	Walk 20 min.	REST

"Am I ready to move to the next phase?" If all is well, you are ready for phase 3. Congratulations! If you're not comfortable, repeat the 8-week phase 2 program until you can comfortably walk 20 minutes, 5 days a week.

Phase 3: Weekly Lifestyle

Is this YOU? "I've successfully worked through phase 2." Or "I've been walking consistently three times a week for 20 to 30 minutes." If you need more of a challenge, maybe phase 4 would better suit your activity level.

Goal: To work towards walking the equivalent of 30 minutes per day almost every day.

	CHALLENGE	DAY 1	DAY 2	DAY 3	DAY 4	DAY 5	DAY 6	DAY 7
WK 1	Stick to it!	Walk 20 min.	Walk 30 min.	Walk 40 min.	REST	Walk 20 min.	Walk 30 min.	Walk 40 min.
WK 2	Take a day off if you need to	Walk 20 min.	Walk 30 min.	Walk 40 min.	REST	Walk 20 min.	Walk 30 min.	Walk 40 min.

This program fits with the American College of Sports Medicine's recommendation of 30 minutes of walking almost every day. Continue with this weekly pattern, walking 20 to 40 minutes almost every day. Enjoy your new, active lifestyle!

"Am I ready to move to the next phase?" Please know that you can be happy with this level of activity without ever feeling you must try to do more. However, if you'd like to try to walk farther, you are ready for phase 4.

Phase 4: Doing More

Is this YOU? "I've successfully worked through phase 3." Or "I'm an avid walker and comfortable walking the equivalent of 30 minutes a day almost every day."

Goal: To work towards walking up to 60 minutes once in a while, a distance of about 3 miles (5 kilometers).

	CHALLENGE	DAY 1	DAY 2	DAY 3	DAY 4	DAY 5	DAY 6	DAY 7
WK 1	Building	Walk 20 min.	Walk 30 min.	Walk 40 min.	REST	Walk 30 min.	Walk 40 min.	Walk 50 min.
WK 2	Progressing further	Walk 30 min.	Walk 40 min.	Walk 50 min.	REST	Walk 30 min.	Walk 40 min.	Walk 50 min.
WK 3	I like the distance	Walk 20 min.	Walk 30 min.	Walk 40 min.	REST	Walk 30 min.	Walk 40 min.	Walk 60 min.
WK 4	Recovery	Walk 20 min.	Walk 30 min.	Walk 40 min.	REST	Walk 20 min.	Walk 30 min.	Walk 40 min.

At this stage, you are ready to make your own decisions. You may decide you like the variety in this 4-week cycle and choose to repeat it, or you may decide to create your own pattern, choosing your own daily walking distances, depending on your route and how you feel. To maintain this phase, walk anywhere between 20 and 60 minutes at a time, and remember to include some variety to help prevent injury and keep your program interesting.

"Am I ready to move to the next phase?" Please know that you may never wish to go beyond this phase and that you can give yourself a break and go back to phase 3 at any time. If you'd still like to do even more walking, you are ready for the InTraining to Walk 10 Kilometers program (see appendix D).

Warming Up

You need to prepare your body for exercise. Muscles are less efficient when they're cold and are more easily injured, because they lack the flow of blood needed to work. Before you begin your walking session, it's important to spend about 8 to 10 minutes doing a general body warm-up. During phase 1 of the program, warm up with 5 minutes of easy body stretches. Walk at an easy pace and gently move your arms, legs and trunk continuously to get the blood flowing faster. Once warm, stretch your muscles with a slow, controlled sequence of exercises (see appendix A).

Cooling Down

The cool-down portion of your walk is simply a gradual reduction in the pace and intensity of your walk. If you've been walking at a brisk pace, for example, you will need to slow yourself to a comfortable pace. If you've been walking at a comfortable pace, you will want to reduce your intensity to an easy pace. The point is to not suddenly stop walking at the end of your walking session. A good cool-down means remaining active for about 10 to 15 minutes to slowly reduce your heart rate. According to the experts at the American College of Sports Medicine, during your cool-down your goal is to lower your heart rate and breathing rate, which assist with your overall recovery following your walking session.

Walking in hot weather

In hot weather conditions, breathable, lightweight garments are the key to comfort. Some technical clothing fabrics these days are so light and airy you'll feel as if you're sporting your birthday suit. Although some fabrics even offer built-in ultraviolet protection, make sure you apply sunscreen to areas that are not protected by your clothing, such as your face, ears and neck.

Increasing your flexibility

One of the best times to work on your flexibility is after you've cooled down. Your muscles are still warm, which makes it a safe time to extend the length of your stretch. For detailed stretching instructions for engaging the larger walking muscles, such as calves, hamstrings, quadriceps and back, turn to appendix A.

The stretch portion of the cool-down should take 8 to 10 minutes and consist of stretches that are "static," which means little movement. All the muscles used during your walk require a gentle (painless) stretch and should be "held" for anywhere from 20 seconds to 3 minutes.

WALKER PROFILE

Joe and June-Ann

Joe and June-Ann are a husband-and-wife team who took up walking in their mid-sixties. As parents of five active children, they were always big supporters of their kids' love for athletics, driving to all of their various sports activities. Joe and June-Ann only became walkers after retiring to the west coast a few years ago. They had spent most of their adult life on the prairies, where the winters are long and cold, too cold for most people to walk outdoors.

After they had settled into their west coast community, they both found the magnificent ocean views and forest trails inspired their initial interest in walking. They loved exploring their new community on foot. The only problem was their lack of fitness—it restricted the trails they were able to explore and the distance they could cover. After talking with their daughter Lynn about their desire to walk more, she encouraged them to join a walking clinic.

Joe and June-Ann signed up for a Learn to Walk 10 Kilometers group and have never looked back. Now into the second year, the two walkers love the structure of the three to four weekly walks as well as the company and energy the group provides. Initially, they were a little tired from the increased demands of a regular training program, but before long they were comfortable with both the distance and speed of the weekly walks. These days, when Joe and June-Ann are not walking with their group, they are exploring neighboring communities and breathing in the west coast air they love so much.

Finding Your Walking Pace

Your walking pace is the speed at which you can comfortably walk. It's not important how fast you walk, but it will take time to get to know your body, and too often beginners take the approach that exercise has to hurt in order for it to work. But in the early stages of your walking program it's much better to walk too slowly than too quickly. Walking at an overly aggressive pace can lead to fatigue and possibly injury.

As you become fitter and stronger, you'll want to get your heart working and make walking a cardiovascular activity. To do this, you need to walk at a brisk pace. This is not a slow jaunt during which you can take in all the sights and sounds of the outdoors. Walking briskly means that you can speak at least two consecutive sentences without huffing and puffing, but you should be breathing heavily after speaking about four to five consecutive sentences. If you're out of breath after speaking a couple of sentences, you need to reduce your speed. Don't be discouraged throughout this process—finding the right pace takes practice.

Good Walking Techniques

There is no such thing as a wrong way to walk, but you can certainly separate the graceful from the ungainly walking form. By incorporating good technique, you will engage your core (stomach and back) muscles, increase your speed and become a more efficient walker. Changing your form may feel awkward at first, but with a little practice you will soon feel as though you're floating along the path.

Talk test

By giving yourself the talk test while exercising, you can easily establish whether you're exercising at your optimal level. If you can speak two consecutive sentences without gasping for air, you are probably exercising within a suitable aerobic range. If you cannot speak even one sentence without struggling to take a breath, you're likely pushing yourself too hard, and you need to reduce your walking pace.

Find the right pace. An easy pace requires little effort. A *comfortable pace* means you can hold a conversation. A *brisk pace* means you are slightly winded after speaking two consecutive sentences, but if you're huffing and puffing it means you are pushing yourself too hard, and you need to back off.

Stay relaxed

One of the best ways to improve your walking performance and your overall enjoyment is to focus on staying relaxed. At various times throughout your walk, it's a good idea to go through a mental checklist to see if your head, shoulders, arms, hands and hips are relaxed.

Try these tips to walk with good technique:

1. Arms dictate the pace, so make the most of your arm swing, whether you're walking briskly or at a comfortable pace.

2. For a good arm swing, you want your arms to be bent at about 90 degrees, with your hands and fingers relaxed. Your palms should face inward, with the thumbs pointed upward and cutting the air to chest height in front of your body. Allow your arms to swing easily and freely, keeping your elbows bent. As your arms reach their maximum extension behind the body, your thumbs should brush just past the hips.

3. When you're walking at a comfortable pace you should stand nice and tall, with square shoulders and arms swinging freely in an upward and backward motion, and your stride should be wide, with a strong heel-toe motion.

4. When you're walking at a brisk pace, your arm motion is the same as when you're at a comfortable pace, but make a conscious effort to drive the arms forward and back. At a brisk pace, swing your thumbs to shoulder height in front of your body; behind your body, drive the elbows as high as shoulder height so that the thumbs and hands are well past the hips, depending on your comfort and flexibility.

5. During a brisk-paced walk, stand tall and square. When your arms are activated, your legs move with them! With a brisker pace, your torso tips slightly forward, your heel-toe action becomes stronger as the knees straighten and your hips swing left and

right to accommodate the straightened knees and strong heel placement. Think about consciously using the muscles in your buttocks to propel yourself forward. If this sounds complicated, don't worry. This "near race-walking technique" comes naturally when the pace picks up.

Walking up hills

- Lean forward into the hill, starting from your waist.
- Keep your stomach and back muscles taut.
- Focus your eyes only a few feet in front of you (avoid searching for the top of the hill).
- Shorten your stride and use small, quick steps.
- Pump your arms—as always, your arms will dictate the pace.

Dress for the weather

Generally, when you first start your walk you should feel a little bit chilly. Body heat generated through exercise is amazing. Within only a short period of time you will warm up. You might even have to take off your outer layer and wrap it around your waist.

Diana

Diana is a fit and active 62-year-old in excellent health. About 20 years ago, she and her husband became golf enthusiasts and began walking regularly in the winter months in order to stay fit for their new hobby.

Today, Diana walks at least 30 minutes a day, and on weekends she generally does at least one longer walk. Maintaining a regular walking program has provided her with endless benefits. In addition to improving her overall well-being, Diana says, "During the menopausal stage of my life, walking had a huge impact on my sleep patterns. On the days where I had played 18 holes of golf, I always slept like a log, but if I didn't walk or only completed a short walk, I would then have sleepless nights." Once Diana realized the correlation, on the days that she didn't play golf she started to increase the duration of her walks and found that she had few sleep problems.

Diana lives in a snowy climate but still manages to walk, even during the coldest days of winter. She prefers to walk alone or with her husband. To keep her walks interesting, Diana likes to observe the different vegetation and watch as the trees and plants change and grow with each passing season. On longer walks, she often explores new housing developments in her city—she finds that walking is a great way to get outside, enjoy the fresh air and stay fit while remaining connected to her community.

Focus on rolling through your foot and pushing off with the balls of your feet.

- Be patient with yourself; it will take time to build your strength and confidence. After a few hills, you will begin to feel stronger and you'll love the feeling of reaching the top!

Encouraging Words from Experienced Walkers

Start slowly: By following your training schedule, you will be properly guided so that you avoid doing too much too soon. Make your goals long-term ones. Remember that it takes time to learn to walk regularly.

Go at your own pace: If you're walking with a partner or a group, don't be pressured into going too fast just to

Gerard

Gerard has always been a big man. Now 47 years old, close to 500 pounds (227 kilograms) and at 5 feet 5 inches (165 centimeters), he feels noticeably larger than all of his family, friends and colleagues. A few months ago, he noticed his coworkers watching whenever he took out his lunch. He was certain he heard snickers whenever he walked by their desks. He felt so self-conscious that he requested permission to telecommute 3 days a week. He reasoned that it was better for the environment if he only drove to the office twice a week. Although Gerard felt more at ease at home, he also realized that his long-term health was at greater risk: he was more sedentary than at work, and he was free to eat whenever and whatever he wanted.

Last Christmas, Gerard's sister, Rachel, gave him a book on walking for exercise. On the inside cover Rachel wrote that if he wanted, she would meet him three mornings a week for a 30-minute walk. At first, Gerard would walk on a small, circular path for a few minutes, then rest on a bench. While he rested, his sister continued walking and circled back to pick him up. For the first time in his life he had fun while exercising. Before long, Gerard could complete a 3-mile (5-kilometer) walk with Rachel. He loved the fresh air and was proud of the changes he had made. He was also surprised by the connection between exercise and diet: the more he walked, the more he wanted to eat well. In 7 months, he lost 60 pounds (27 kilograms) and felt better than he had in years.

Walking for Fitness

keep up. If you set out a route beforehand so that everyone knows where you'll finish the walk, you won't have to be concerned about dropping back and walking on your own.

Stick with the plan: Try not to miss a session. If you do, don't try to make it up by doing double the next time. Consistent training works best. Using a set program takes the guesswork out of achieving fitness.

Learn from others: Experience is the best teacher. Learn from talking and sharing with others who walk regularly, such as a training partner or those in your walking group.

Think positively: Focus on what feels good, not on what hurts. At the beginning of the program, there will be various aches and pains that develop as your body begins to adapt to the new stress levels. Be patient; this is all part of the process.

Find a friend: Especially for those longer walks, try to buddy up with someone. It sure helps to know that someone is on the corner waiting for you, and you can push and pull each other through the session.

Talk to yourself: The farther you go in the training process, the easier it gets. There is always a reason not to go out and exercise, but the reasons to exercise are always better. Persevere with the program. Remind yourself that it will get easier! As your fitness increases, so will your self-esteem and confidence.

Make time to walk: Plan to exercise at a time that is most convenient for you. Some people like to get up early and start the day with their exercise regime. Others

i Rainy-day walking

In rainy conditions, a baseball-style hat is a must. Ideally, the hat should be waterproof. If you've never worn hats or don't like them, give one a try—you'll be amazed at how much more you enjoy walking in the rain.

fit it in during their lunch hour or sometime after work. The point is to schedule and protect your walking time so that it doesn't get taken up with other demands.

Congratulate yourself: After a good workout, stop and think about how great you feel. Remember how that felt, so that the next time you're not too keen about heading out, you can look forward to how fantastic you will feel after.

The Psychology of Exercise

MIND OVER MATTER. FINDING THE COURAGE TO MAKE exercise a part of your daily routine is not an easy task. The physical demands alone can be overwhelming. But equally important are the mental demands. Motivation, commitment and perseverance are factors that can help, hinder and even sideline your fitness goals. From information on the science behind the postexercise "high" to guidelines for maneuvering your way through the motivational potholes common to any exercise program, this chapter provides you with everything you will need to know to take your first, second and third steps down the road to improved health and fitness.

The Psychological Benefits of Walking

You may be asking yourself, "If it's so difficult to start and maintain an exercise program, how do people find the commitment to stick with it?" The answer is easy: it feels good. Psychological researchers Dr. Jerrold S. Greenberg and Dr. David Pargman have spent years studying the interrelationship between body and mind. They say that the five components of health are mental, physical, emotional,

The psychological benefits of walking

- positively affects memory and concentration
- improves mood and feeling of well-being
- decreases anxiety and stress levels
- improves self-confidence and body image

social and spiritual. Each one influences the others, therefore making good health dependent on the balance between the five elements.

The exerciser's "high"

If you know any people who run, chances are you have had the occasion to hear them boast of their postexercise "high." Or maybe you've seen the smiles and heard the elated chatter of cyclists after a long ride; in this mind-set, it's almost as if they could conquer anything. "Calm," "clear" and at times "euphoric" are the words commonly used to describe it. The positive state of mind that reportedly follows most extended exercise sessions is often referred to as the "runner's high," but don't be fooled into believing that runners have cornered the market on postexercise euphoria. This state of mind can be captured after a good walk or any other form of exercise that's done over an extended period of time.

The "runner's high" is immeasurable, because it is a concept based completely on personal experience. However, exercise-science researchers tell us that endorphins, the body's natural painkillers, are released during lengthy or strenuous exercise and can lead to improved mood and general feelings of happiness. Health care professionals will often encourage patients to take up a regular exercise program as a wellness activity that can prevent emotional distress and potentially improve a healthy individual's resistance to disease.

Commonly Asked Questions about the Psychology of Walking

Q. *Can walking improve my ability to cope with stress?*

A. Yes. Regular exercise helps to reduce anxiety and decrease chronic and daily stress, thus contributing to mental health and well-being. As well, exercise is a way of getting rid of tension or pent-up frustration. It's also thought that exercise provides individuals with a distraction from the pressures and anxieties of daily living. For some of you, a daily walk might be the only time in the day when you are removed from the demands of work and family obligations. So, the next time your mind feels frazzled, take a walk around the block. You'll likely find that your tense muscles will gradually relax, leaving you calmer and happier at the end of your walk.

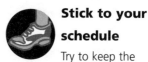

Stick to your schedule

Try to keep the appointment you made with yourself and do your walking workout at a time of day that works best for you. Whatever time of day you choose, it's most important to make your walking session a priority.

WALKER PROFILE

Kahram

Kahram is 57 years old and has been playing golf for more than 30 years. He usually plays four to five times a week, walking for close to 5 hours while carrying a 40-pound (18-kilogram) golf bag on his shoulder. Kahram finds that his passion for golf keeps him fit. He says, "Every golf course is different. The variety of different courses as well as the substantial green fees keep me motivated to stay fit. In order for me to enjoy the game, I need to play to the best of my ability." In the past, he's found that if he's unfit, his breathing is labored at the start of each hole, which means less energy and little focus. All of this leads to bad golf scores, which makes Kahram unhappy.

When Kahram isn't playing golf, he's busy with the small doughnut shop he and his son, Bud, have run for over 10 years. The two work side by side most mornings making the doughnuts for the morning rush. After things slow down, Kahram attends to the numerous administrative duties of the business, including walking to the many meetings he has outside the restaurant. Not only is doing the bulk of his errands without a car more efficient for Kahram, it gives him a reason to walk, is better for the environment and helps him maintain his fitness for the golf course.

i Be confident

You can do this! Hold your head high. Keep your body proud, tall and upright. Focus on your arms. LIFT those knees immediately after your feet hit the ground, and plant your heel firmly with each step. Breathe comfortably and naturally, and concentrate your gaze just ahead of you. Feel good and look good for all to see!

i Reward yourself

You've worked hard and deserve a new, peppy item of clothing for walking! If you've been walking for a while, treat yourself to a new shirt that will wick moisture away from your body, leave you drier than your cotton T-shirt and provide more comfort during your workout. You'll look and feel better when you walk.

Q. *Does walking alleviate depression?*

A. Depression should not be approached lightly, so if you are depressed or know someone who is, you need to seek advice from a health care professional. Most practitioners who treat patients with mild or moderate depression usually recommend exercise as part of the treatment. It is accepted by most of the health science community that general mood elation commonly follows exercise. For these effects to be long term, you must maintain a regular and consistent fitness schedule.

Q. *How much do I need to walk before I can receive the psychological benefits?*

A. Surprisingly, fitness research shows that short walks of no more than 10 minutes can help to lower tension, sadness and anxiety and improve your overall mood.

Q. *Why are fit people generally happy with their body size and shape?*

A. For the most part, fit folks who exercise regularly have a better body image than people who are sedentary. Studies show that individuals who maintain a consistent exercise regime will, over time, begin to see positive physical changes in their bodies. Once a person sees these positive results, it often triggers a variety of positive responses, including healthy eating habits, as well as improved self-confidence and body image.

Train Your Mind

It takes mental strength and fortitude to stay on track with a regular fitness routine. Maintaining focus and motivation is challenging for the most seasoned athlete. Trust that there will be days when you will not feel like walking—curling up in front of the fire with a good book and a mug of hot chocolate will be more enticing than hitting the cold, wet streets for a 30-minute walk. Keep in mind that you're not alone—everyone, regardless of age or fitness level, experiences dips in motivation. Each of us has days when getting out for a walk seems an insurmountable challenge; however, use the suggestions in this chapter to help you overcome some of the common mental barriers to exercise.

Plan a program that meets your goals

Your doctor may have told you that you need to exercise and that a walking program would be a good start. The programs and advice in this book will provide you with the tools to create a walking plan that meets your needs.

Set short- and long-term goals

It's extremely important, especially if you're feeling discouraged, to establish both short- and long-term fitness goals that are realistic for you. For example, your short-term goal could be to walk around your apartment for a few minutes today, and your long-term quest could be to walk to your local grocery store and back. The point is for you to experience small successes that will reconfirm your commitment to an active lifestyle.

Build your confidence step-by-step

You may feel intimidated or self-conscious about exercising in front of others. Trying a new skill or activity

 Fitness consultant Diana Rochon of Whistler, B.C., suggests the following strategies for overcoming mental barriers common to beginning exercisers:

Planning: Find a program you simply follow every day.

Confidence: Trust that once you start the program and discover you can do it, your anxieties will diminish.

Commitment: Be realistic with the program you choose, using both doable short-term and long-term goals. When you see small successes daily, you'll be more likely to stick with it.

Support: Include the help of those who love you the most. This support is essential to your success and enjoyment.

can be daunting the first few times, but after a while the activity is no longer new and your anxiety may slowly disappear. Until you become comfortable with your new fitness regime, it's okay to find a less populated park or a quiet street on which to start your walking program. For safety reasons, walk with a dog or just let someone know where you are.

Commit to your walking program

At first glance, walking appears simple. After all, you've been doing it for most of your life. But if you haven't exercised in a while and you grow tired quickly after walking a short distance, you may be extremely discouraged. It's important to know that you're not alone. As Dr. Bryan Barootes points out in chapter 2, the first step for some people will be moving around the house for a couple of minutes at a time. After all, everyone has to start somewhere, and while you might be unhappy with your current fitness level, if you start walking today, you are that much closer to being the fit person you want to become.

Enlist the support of others

Too often, people new to exercise try to do it alone, without the support of their family members and friends. It may seem like a secret endeavor that you want to do on your own, but including the help of those who love you the most is essential to your success and enjoyment. Once these folks know you're committed to your fitness goals, the chances are good that they will do everything they can to support you along the way to improved health and fitness. And don't be surprised if you inspire one or two of them to join you.

Goal Setting

You've likely heard it said before that a goal is like a dream with a date on it. Knowing what direction you want to go is a sign that you are taking some control of your future. Most people, regardless of how smart, fit or fantastic they are, do not achieve success in anything without doing some planning and goal setting. To minimize and avoid setbacks with a new walking program, Dr. Whitney Sedgwick, a Vancouver psychologist who works in the sports realm, encourages people to avoid setting goals that are overly vague, unrealistic or not meaningful enough to the person. To maximize your chances of success with your new walking program, Dr. Sedgwick suggests setting specific goals that are realistic and meaningful. Setting specific goals allows you to measure your progress/success and feel good about it; setting realistic goals (no matter how small) means that you have a good chance of achieving them and building your confidence, and setting meaningful goals will motivate you to stick with your program even if you encounter setbacks along the way.

Establish your walking goals

Success depends on motivation and goal setting. Desire, values and beliefs are the three factors that motivate you to take action and act the way you do. Desire means the goal is an unsatisfied longing you wish to satisfy; value means you attach importance to it, and belief is when

i Do an out-and-back walk that takes you from a starting point to a turnaround destination and back to your starting point. This kind of walk is motivating, because once you reach the turnaround point, you know that you are halfway to the finish line of your session, and staying focused is always easier on the way home.

you are of the opinion that the goal has meaning. You have control of your beliefs, values and desires, which means if you attach value and see them as important, you are more likely to successfully motivate yourself. When you combine internal motivation with realistic goals, your chances of success drastically increase.

Before you set your walking goals, record on a piece of paper or in a walking journal your answers to the following three questions:

1. What desires, beliefs and values do you attach to walking and fitness in general? For example, "I believe walking will help to improve my health and fitness, which will improve the likelihood of living a long and healthy life." Set a goal for yourself, such

Sarah

Sarah is a 47-year-old graphic designer whose first husband died in a tragic car accident that left her shattered. She knew instinctively that she would never get over her loss, but as a way of coping with it, Sarah began to walk at night. She had always been a runner, and she continued to run most mornings before work, but the evenings became her time for walking.

Every night after dinner, Sarah would head out for a long walk along the river near her apartment. It was cold and windy during the winter and muggy during the summer, but she welcomed the extreme conditions—they were a distraction from her darkness. For Sarah, walking became meditative and therapeutic, a time during which she felt most at peace in the world. She was alone with her sadness, yet somehow felt less alone than when she was with family and friends or at home in her apartment. As the years passed, her grief seemed to lessen and her desire to walk for extended periods of time diminished.

When Sarah first met her second husband, Phil, she told him about her walks; being a police officer, he expressed concern for her safety. She understood his worries, but she covets this time and took offense when Phil suggested that she take up an indoor hobby. Today he is still concerned for his wife's safety, but he is comforted that she allows their new border collie puppy, Thursday, to join her on most of her walks.

Walking for Fitness

as "I will work towards achieving phase 1 of the walking program."

2. What are your strengths and weaknesses in maintaining a fitness program? For example, "I am good at starting an exercise program, but after a while it takes a backseat to my work and family responsibilities. If I could somehow have my partner join me in my walking plans, I would be better able to stick with a program." A possible goal might be: "I will ask my partner to join me on tonight's walk."

3. What are some of the barriers you perceive to your achieving your walking goals? For example, "I work long hours and have family responsibilities, which make it difficult to find the time to walk." A possible goal: "I will walk for 10 minutes during my lunch hour." Or "I will walk to work twice a week."

By writing down your responses to these three questions, you are creating a workable plan and reinforcing your commitment to your goals. Social science researchers indicate that people who record their goals are more committed than those who do not and are more likely to achieve a successful outcome. Once you have a clear understanding of your strengths and weaknesses and the potential pitfalls you face in achieving an active lifestyle, you will be better prepared to set realistic and achievable goals.

Set different types of goals

Although you may have one overall goal—to become fitter or to walk 6 miles (10 kilometers), for example—having various related goals can help you to maintain your focus and motivation. Including a variety of goals, like the ones below, provides you with numerous options for monitoring and measuring your success. Consider incorporating the following goals into your own walking plan:

- *Lifestyle:* Lifestyle goals are directed towards your way of living or daily life. For example, "I will no longer eat snacks that are high in fat and sugar after dinner; instead I will go for a 15-minute walk."
- *Outcome:* Outcome goals are centered around your anticipated results. For example, "By the end of my 13-week walking program, I will be able to walk 3 miles (5 kilometers) in 90 minutes, which will be a personal best for me."
- *Process:* Process goals focus on your ongoing performance and can be physical, psychological or technical. For example, "During tonight's walk I will focus only on the positive aspects about myself. I will not allow myself any negative self-talk regarding my weight management issues."
- *Social:* Social goals are centered on community or the company of others. For example, "I will go for a walk with my son every weekend."
- *Time:* "I will walk four times a week for 30 minutes."

Be realistic with your goals

It will take time for your body to adjust to the increased demands of your new walking lifestyle. Change takes time and so does incorporating positive habits. It's essential that you create positive associations with your walking. If you experience only feelings of ambivalence

Walking for Fitness

or dread every time you think about going for a walk, it's unlikely that you will stay on the right track to achieving your goals. By setting realistic goals for yourself from the outset, you will be more likely to train your mind and your body at the same time. By experiencing small successes along the way, before long you will begin to see yourself as a person who walks and someone who exercises regularly. This new attitude will build your confidence and your enjoyment in walking. Once you enjoy your new activity, you are more likely to stick with it.

Make Walking a Habit

Walking is like any other aspect of your life: once it becomes a habit or a pattern, similar to flossing your teeth at night or taking out the recycling bins on Wednesday mornings, your chances of sticking with it and achieving your walking goals significantly increase. Dr. Sedgwick says that establishing habits and routines around your walking program from the start increases your chances of maintaining your new active lifestyle.

Don't be overly concerned if it takes you a while to figure out the right formula for success. Determining when and where you should walk as well as whether you prefer walking in solitude or in the company of a friend can be a process of trial and error. These factors will quickly work themselves out if you are flexible and open to different ideas. If this is a new endeavor, it's important to have fun with it. Once you find something that works, repeat it, and before long you will have created your own routine.

 Sport psychologist Dr. Whitney Sedgwick suggests that most goals need to be:

- as specific and as concise as possible
- measurable, so that you know you are moving towards your goal
- adjustable and modifiable, if needed
- realistic and appropriate for you
- time based, so that you are working around a deadline
- exciting for you, so that you see your goal as something you want to achieve
- in writing, so that you can check your own goals regularly

Understanding change

Change does not occur overnight and it's not always easy—it takes time, patience and commitment. As part of their study of how people behave, American social science researchers Dr. James O. Prochaska and Dr. Carlo C. DiClemente have created the "transtheoretical" model of change. This five-stage model explains the mental shifts that people must make in order to change a behavior:

Stage 1
Pre-contemplation is when there is little or no desire to change.
Stage 2
Contemplation occurs when an individual sees that there is a negative pattern or habit that exists and is considering how he or she might change.
Stage 3
Preparation is when a person is ready to take action to change the problem behavior.
Stage 4
Action happens when an individual addresses the problem, implements more positive behaviors and creates an environment that supports the change.
Stage 5
Maintenance is when work is done to minimize chances of slipping back into previous patterns.

Be an optimist

Social science research suggests that the key difference separating people who can change successfully from those who cannot is the ability to believe in oneself. Those who are confident are generally optimistic regarding their ability to cope with a wide variety of situations, whereas those who are less confident are prone to more anxiety, are less optimistic about their ability to control certain events in their lives, and therefore have a limited belief in themselves.

Seeing yourself in a new way is going to take time, especially if you've been sedentary for most of your life or if you have been active in the past but now struggle with weight management issues. With a gradual and progressive walking plan and a good dose of old-fashioned patience and commitment, you can change and become a fit and healthy person.

Set small, realistic goals

"Slow and steady wins the race" might be a tired old adage, but it's stood the test of time for a reason: it's true. It's tempting for many beginning walkers to do too much too soon. When this happens it's easy to experience feelings of failure, which can make a person retreat into old habits. Remember, to increase your self-confidence and self-belief you need to set small, realistic goals. By regularly experiencing incremental accomplishments you begin to feel what it's like to be successful, which will in turn increase your confidence and the belief you have in your ability to achieve your goals.

Be gentle with yourself

Motivation to exercise is like any other area of your life: there are bound to be ebbs and flows. There will be days when all you can do is to make it to the end of your day so that you can get outside and enjoy the peacefulness of your evening walk. But there will be other times when it's a struggle just to put on your walking shoes. Dr. Sedgwick encourages beginning exercisers to understand that it's impossible to be 100 percent motivated to exercise all the time. Everyone has busy lives with competing demands, so it's understandable that when you've been up most of the night caring for a sick child, you will have less energy and therefore less motivation to walk. For the most part, you want your motivation to be as consistent as possible while still cutting yourself some slack. Here are some suggestions for keeping yourself motivated:

- *Solidify your commitment:* List some of the reasons you want to become a person who walks regularly. Writing them down will force you to think about what this new habit represents in your life. It will also increase your personal commitment to becoming a person who walks.

- *Make your goals known:* Post your list of reasons in an easy-to-read location such as on your fridge or in your daily planner.

- *Engage in positive self-talk:* When you're walking or thinking about walking, try to talk to yourself in a positive manner, and remind yourself that each day you're getting stronger, healthier and fitter.

- *Write down some motivating words:* Write a list of key words that you can repeat during a difficult part of your walk. It doesn't matter what words you choose; they just need to evoke positive feelings for you, such as those evoked by the phrases "smooth and graceful" or "strong and agile."

- *Celebrate your successes:* Reward yourself after small and large achievements. By treating yourself to a hot bubble bath or by taking a friend for coffee, you are marking your achievement and reinforcing the value you place on your health and fitness.

- *Maintain focus:* Only focus on one walk at a time—don't worry about a previously scheduled walk that you missed or the one at the end of the week. Just think about the one that you'll do today.

- *Paint a picture:* Create a picture in your mind of yourself already succeeding, such as crossing the finish line of a 6-mile (10-kilometer) event with your hands in the air and a smile on your face.

WALKER PROFILE

Lisa

Lisa is a 52-year-old stay-at-home mom. She was a competitive runner during her university days and ran professionally before she met her husband and began having children. As an elite athlete, Lisa's first passion was running, but she always used walking as a way to relax and to recover from hard runs. As well, she often used walking as a means of transportation.

These days, when Lisa is not shuttling her five kids to school, soccer or ballet, she tries to do a 30-minute leisurely run a few times a week. She also does some freelance sports writing for an online publication. While researching an article, she learned that there is an increasing demand for pedometers, instruments that calculate the approximate distance traveled on foot by counting the number of steps taken. Lisa was curious about her own average number of steps and purchased a pedometer. She was shocked to find that on the days she didn't run, she walked fewer than 2,000 steps. Her research suggested that the average sedentary person walks between 1,000 and 3,000 steps per day.

Lisa realized that she depended more on a car than on her feet, and she started to consider the impact on her kids. Her children all played sports at least twice a week, but otherwise they were driven everywhere. Lisa decided to begin walking to as many of her errands as possible. As well, she began walking her kids to school. Initially they complained, but before long they started to enjoy being outside, laughing and being together as family. On the weekends, they often walk with their dad to rent movies or to buy special treats at the grocery store for Saturday night.

Borrow a pedometer

For one day, pay attention to the number of steps you take. You'll likely discover you are a far cry from the recommended 10,000 daily steps, so much so that it will reconfirm your commitment to walk more.

Keep a journal or logbook

Training journals or logbooks are places where you record the details of your exercise program. You could record: the date, route, effort, days you might be sick or injured and unable to do your exercise, and the total distance or duration of the walk, as well as the weekly and monthly distance or time totals. Dr. Barootes encourages his patients who take up a walking program to keep a journal recording the type, time and duration of activity. He also suggests that you keep track of your overall response to each session, such as enjoyment or discomfort, so that you can reflect on your progress and achievements. It may also assist in identifying factors that contribute to any problems (especially overuse injuries) that you may encounter.

A walking journal can be a good motivator if you get burned out or bored and want to quit after a few weeks of walking. As well, it's a great tool to analyze the effects of your training, monitor progress, establish ways to improve your walking plan and avoid injury.

Slip on a pedometer

If you want to get a clear sense of your activity level, you might try slipping on a pedometer first thing in the morning before you get up and take it off before you go to sleep. A pedometer is an instrument that looks much like a pager, only it's used to record the distance a person covers on foot. The instrument is specifically designed to respond to the body motion of each step. A pedometer clips onto the waistband of your pants to detect the movements from walking that cause your hips to move up and down.

Research shows that people who walk 10,000 steps (about 5 miles/8 kilometers) every day can reduce their chances of developing coronary heart disease, minimize high blood pressure and more easily manage a healthy body weight. Once you know the number of steps you take on an average day, you can decide for yourself if you need to add more movement to become more active. At the end of the day, your pedometer reading is concrete proof that fitness is about an accumulation of activity over the course of a day, week, month and year. It shows you that if you don't have time to take 30 minutes from your busy schedule for a brisk walk, there are numerous other ways to meet your daily step goal.

Engage in positive self-talk

Cheerleading and positive self-talk alone do not give you the ability to believe in yourself and change old habits. They do, however, play a significant role in the process. You cannot believe in yourself and your ability to change while maintaining an inner dialogue that you're a lazy, good-for-nothing fool! Instead of ignoring negative thoughts, positive thinkers are able to admit when they feel frustrated or unhappy. Not only do they acknowledge these thoughts, they try to understand why they are feeling a certain way and figure out a plan to move into a more positive mind-set. Staying positive is not easy, especially if you have recent experience with failure or frustration. As you embark on your new walking program, try to recognize that each time you make it out the door for a walk, it's an achievement. An active lifestyle is a journey to be enjoyed, one step at a time.

What to look for in a pedometer

The Canadian Health Network provides the following tips for buying a pedometer. It should:
- count steps accurately
- have a cover to protect the display
- include a belt clip or strap so the pedometer doesn't fall off when you wear it
- use an inexpensive battery (such as a watch battery)

You can find pedometers at most large drugstores and athletic shops.

Fueling the Body

"Every single organ system, bone tissue and cell in your body benefits from good nutrition. It is a wise investment wih a huge return on your quality of life."
—Jennifer Gibson, registered sport dietitian

AS A PERSON WHO EXERCISES REGULARLY, FUELING YOUR body with good food can mean the difference between a brisk walk that feels as though your feet hardly touched the ground and a never-ending shuffle that leaves you exhausted and discouraged at the end of your workout. Good nutrition will help your performance, boost your energy levels and aid the recovery and repair of your muscles.

Fueling for Exercise

There's an overwhelming amount of information available on healthy eating and special diets promising to give you the body you deserve in a matter of weeks. But the truth of the matter is that when it comes to healthy eating, the basics are all you need to know to get you on the right track.

The Three Rights
R: The *Right* Food
R: The *Right* Amount
R: The *Right* Time

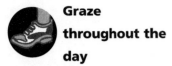 **Graze throughout the day**

Avoid going longer than 4 hours during the day without eating. When exercising, it's a good idea to eat BEFORE you feel hungry; when not exercising, try to limit your eating to when you're hungry, and chew slowly to give your body time to register that it's full.

Stock your kitchen with the following foods to ensure that you have a variety of foods for preparing healthy and tasty meals:

The right food

A healthy diet essentially means eating a variety of foods from the four main food groups: grains, breads and cereals; fruits and vegetables; meat and alternatives; milk and other calcium sources. By striving to eat within these guidelines you will give your body the vitamins, minerals and nutrients it needs to be healthy, strong and energized throughout the day. As well, Vancouver-based registered dietitian Jennifer Gibson, who specializes in sport nutrition, says that the goal of a healthy diet should be to include three meals a day and two to three snacks. The largest portion of your food should come from vegetables or fruit and some protein.

Food Group	Function	Foods to Choose
Grains, breads and cereals	Energy. Grains contain carbohydrates, which are the body's preferred fuel source. Seventy percent of the brain runs on glycogen, which is the storage form of carbohydrate in the body. This is what is fueling your body while you are walking! B vitamins are found in fortified grain products and are responsible for energy metabolism in the body. Fiber, which is found in these foods, contributes to bowel regularity and may reduce the risk of heart disease and some cancers.	Whole wheat breads, pitas, bagels and rolls; whole wheat pastas, noodles and rice; high-fiber hot and cold cereals.

Walking for Fitness

Food Group	Function	Foods to Choose
Fruits and vegetables	Fruits and vegetables contain a range of vitamins and minerals that are responsible for all of the cellular reactions that keep the body functioning. They also contain fiber and carbohydrates for energy. They protect against the effects of aging and reduce the risk of cancer and heart disease.	Dark green, orange, yellow and red fruits and vegetables; canned and frozen vegetables.
Meat and meat alternatives	Meats and meat alternatives contain powerful protein and minerals such as iron. Protein is responsible for the repair and recovery of the muscle tissue in the body. Our immune cells, hair, skin and nails are also made from protein. Fish, nuts and seeds contain healthy fats called mono- and polyunsaturates. These fats play a critical role in our cellular health and can also lower the risk of heart disease.	Lean meats such as beef, pork, chicken and fish; tofu; eggs; peanut butter, nuts and seeds; beans (black, kidney, et cetera).
Milk and calcium sources	These foods contain calcium and other minerals essential for bone health. Calcium is also responsible for regulation of cellular functions such as muscle contraction.	Calcium-fortified soy beverages and foods; milk; cheese; yogurt.

Healthy eating can be quick and simple

- Try marinated raw vegetables for an afternoon snack. Put some asparagus stalks into a resealable plastic bag, add low-calorie Italian dressing and let them marinate for 30 minutes.

- Freeze a piece of steak in a resealable plastic bag. Remove it from the freezer the night before you plan to eat it, add your favorite barbecue sauce right into the bag and let it marinate and defrost in the refrigerator overnight.

You may have noticed that "sweets and treats" like fast foods, cakes, doughnuts and potato chips are not among the recommended foods. From a nutrition point of view, these foods have little to offer in the way of vitamins, minerals and fiber. For the most part, these foods are high in fat and sugar and are therefore empty calories. They don't provide you with the essential nutrients you need, and while they may taste great initially, they can actually hinder your health and your fitness experience.

This is not to say that you should deprive yourself of the occasional treat; you just want to eat them in moderation. A reasonable goal is to aim for the 80/20 rule of nutrition. Try to choose healthy options 80 percent of the time, but leave yourself a 20 percent margin for soul foods that offer pure pleasure. After all, no one eats perfectly all the time, and if you know that you're allowed to have the occasional treat, you will look forward to it and savor it more fully than if you ate it often and in large quantities.

The right amount

You now understand what you should eat, but figuring out how much you should eat and when can be difficult, especially when you first become active. Proper fueling before, during and after exercise is an essential component of an active lifestyle, but it's not a straightforward formula. Your height, weight, age, gender and activity level all determine how many calories you need to consume in a day. A calorie is simply the unit of energy obtained from food.

For your body to stay the same weight, the number of calories you consume each day needs to equal the number of calories you burn. Don't forget that you're burning calories all the time, even when you're sitting at a computer or sleeping. If you consume more calories than you burn, they will be stored and eventually become body fat. The reverse is also true; if you take in fewer calories than you burn, you will begin to lose body fat.

The calories-in and calories-out formula is not always a perfect equation, says Jennifer Gibson. As many frustrated dieters can tell you, less food doesn't always equal a thinner body. The body is a smart machine: if it feels it is being deprived of energy, it may go into

Bob

Bob is a 65-year-old retired teacher and the former owner of Mr. C's Pizza. Over the years, teaching, running a small business and coaching his sons' hockey teams didn't leave him very much time for exercise. But after retiring to Arizona with his wife, Bob began cycling and walking most days.

Although Bob had always spent a lot of time on his feet while teaching and operating the busy pizza business, he didn't exercise, and he regularly ate high-fat and sugary foods. In fact, he didn't think about his health until his doctor mentioned the threat of type II diabetes. With a long family history of heart disease, Bob took his doctor's warnings very seriously. He says, "It was as though a light switch went on, and overnight I made the decision to change my diet and begin exercising."

Two years later, 25 pounds (11 kilograms) lighter and a speed walker who clocks 5 miles (8 kilometers) a day, Bob looks back at the changes he made and says he regrets only that he wasn't always as fit. Walking has become a way of life: every day he walks 1¼ miles (2 kilometers) to buy his morning newspaper, then eats a breakfast of hot oatmeal or whole wheat toast as he pores over the sports section. He so enjoys the freedom that fresh air and walking rapidly give him that he's disappointed when forced to take a rest day to recover from a cold or a minor injury. As for his diet, Bob says that once he started walking regularly, his cravings for fat and sugar were drastically reduced, though he still allows himself the odd treat.

Some rules of thumb about portion sizes:

- 1¾–3½ ounces (50–100 grams) of meat = size of a deck of cards
- 1 cup (250 milliliters) of starch = size of a tennis ball or a fist

starvation mode and begin to resist fat loss. The human body evolved this way to be sure it would always have proper fuel, even during times of scarcity. If you want specific weight management suggestions, it's a good idea to seek advice from a registered dietitian, who can assess your needs and make meal planning and recipe suggestions that will work best for you.

The right time

It might seem boring or even a bit obsessive, but if you want to eat in a healthy manner most of the time, you need to plan, plan and plan some more. Ask any individual who has good nutrition and maintains a healthy weight, and chances are that he or she will organize and plan snacks and meals for the upcoming day and possibly even week. Initially, it might seem just another time-consuming task to add to your already busy schedule, but after a while it will become second nature.

Advance planning will help you to eat better and recognize a "mental" hunger that drives many people to overeat. Are you eating because you're bored at work, stressed out about something or because a treat sitting on a friend's counter looks really good? It's important to be aware of what's currently triggering your hunger. Think of your typical day stretched out along a timeline. Plot your exercise and activity and build a meal strategy that will fit. Here are some helpful guidelines:

- Do not go longer than 4 hours without eating.
- Aim to eat at least three-quarters of your food groups at your core meals (breakfast, lunch and dinner).

Walking for Fitness

- Plan one to two snacks throughout the day that contain one to two of the four food groups.
- Drink water with every meal. Try carrying a water bottle with you wherever you go.
- One hour before exercise, eat a high-carbohydrate snack like a granola bar, toast with jelly, or a fruit plus 2 cups (500 mL) of water.
- During exercise, aim for three to four large gulps of water every 15 minutes.
- Within 1 hour after exercise, eat a snack with carbohydrates and protein. Don't forget to drink 2 to 3 cups (500 to 750 mL) of water as well.
- At lunch and dinner, design meals that look like the winning plate below. Half the plate should be vegetables, a quarter starch and a quarter meat, and add a fruit for dessert and a calcium source.

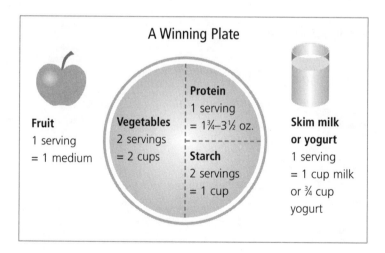

A Winning Plate

Fruit
1 serving
= 1 medium

Vegetables
2 servings
= 2 cups

Protein
1 serving
= 1¾–3½ oz.

Starch
2 servings
= 1 cup

**Skim milk
or yogurt**
1 serving
= 1 cup milk
or ¾ cup
yogurt

Here is an example of a training and nutrition timeline (TNT) for a 59 kg (129 lb.) female recreational walker.

A typical menu for a full day might look something like this:

Meal	Nutrition Goal	Meal Examples
Breakfast 8:00 AM	Aim to have three of the four food groups.	• 1 cup (250 mL) high-fiber cereal + skim milk + medium fruit; • 1 egg + 2 slices whole grain toast + 6 oz. (170 g) yogurt; • 1 cup (250 mL) oatmeal + 10 raisins + chocolate milk
Snack 10:30 AM	Aim to have one to two of the four food groups.	• 4 to 6 medium-sized crackers + 1 tbsp (15 mL) peanut butter; • 6 oz. (170 g) yogurt
Lunch 12:00 PM	Aim to have three to four of the four food groups.	• meat sandwich + 2 cups (500 mL) salad + 1 tbsp (15 mL) low-fat dressing + 6 oz. (170 g) yogurt; • 1½ cups (375 mL) vegetable soup + dinner roll + veggie dog + fruit; • 1 cup (250 mL) veggie chili + 4 to 6 medium-sized crackers + 6 oz. (170 g) yogurt
Pre-walk snack 3:00 PM	Aim to have a carbohydrate + water.	• 1 small fruit + 2 cups (500 mL) water; • ½ an energy bar + 2 cups (500 mL) water
During walk	Water	• three to four gulps of water every 15 minutes
Post-walk snack 6:00 PM	Aim to have a carbohydrate + water.	• 1 small fruit + 2 cups (500 mL) water; • ½ an energy bar + 2 cups (500 mL) water
Dinner 7:00 PM	Aim to have three of the four food groups.	• sushi (8 pieces California roll); • 1 cup (250 mL) rice pasta with meat sauce + 2 cups (500 mL) salad with 1 to 2 tbsp (15 to 30 mL) low-fat dressing; • soy burger on whole wheat bun + 2 cups (500 mL) salad with 1 to 2 tbsp (15 to 30 mL) low-fat dressing; • 1 potato + 1 cup (240 mL) salad with low-fat dressing + 4 oz. (115 g) chicken breast + 6 oz. (170 g) yogurt; • beef stir-fry = 1 cup (250 mL) rice + 1 cup (250 mL) veggies + 2 oz. (57 g) beef

A Word about Weight Management

Weight loss is a challenging endeavor. It is best achieved with a triple-sided approach: healthy eating, exercise and a positive attitude. Successful weight loss is difficult to accomplish on your own. If you're considering a weight loss plan, it's a good idea to make an appointment to see a registered dietitian, who will be able to develop a healthy eating plan that is right for you.

Restricting daily calories too much and/or cutting out entire food groups are recipes for disaster. Unfortunately, there's no safe pill you can take or special diet you can follow that will provide you with lasting results. As dietitian Jennifer Gibson points out, it takes most people a number of months or even years to put on extra weight, so you cannot expect to lose the excess weight in a matter of weeks. Slowly and steadily is the safe and healthy approach to weight management.

Are you at risk?

Getting started on managing your weight means knowing where you are at right now. A good way to do this is to calculate your body mass index (BMI) and waist circumference (WC). The Canadian Guidelines for Body Weight Classification in Adults uses BMI as an indicator of health risk associated with underweight and overweight, and WC as an indicator of health risk associated with abdominal obesity. This classification system applies only to those aged 18 years and over and is not intended for use with women who are pregnant or lactating.

You can calculate your BMI using this formula:

Obesity is a term used to describe a person who has a large amount of body fat. The distinction between an individual who is overweight versus one who is obese usually involves measuring one's body mass index (BMI): one's weight in kilograms divided by the square of one's height in meters. BMI is the measurement of choice for most physicians and researchers studying weight management and obesity.

To measure your body, place a tape measure around your bare abdomen just above the hip bone, using your belly button as a landmark. (The tape measure should cover your belly button.) Be sure the tape is snug but doesn't compress the skin. *Exhale,* relax and measure. Breathe normally and make sure your tape measure is parallel to the floor.

Factors contributing to rising obesity rates are the engineered convenience of the built environment, lack of access to public transit, sedentary jobs, poor access to healthy food choices, and a food-pricing structure that makes the most energy-dense foods (foods high in sugar and unhealthy fats) the cheapest and the healthiest foods the most costly. According to Dr. Diane Finegood of Simon Fraser University, who also is scientific director of the Canadian Institutes of Health Research's Institute of Nutrition, Metabolism and Diabetes in Vancouver, B.C., "We also have to recognize that socioeconomic status plays a role in this enormous challenge. Many people simply haven't the means and/or the wherewithal to purchase healthy, nutritious food."

$$\text{BMI} = \text{weight (kg)} \div \text{height squared (m}^2)$$

To do this, first know your weight in kilograms and height in meters.

Example: 260 lb.; 6 ft.

Weight = 0.454 kg per lb. x 260 lb. = 118 kg

Height = 0.3048 m per ft. x 6 ft. = 1.83 m = 3.35 m^2

BMI = 118 kg $\div$ 3.35 m^2 = 35.2 kg per m^2

(obese class 1)

Health risk classification according to body mass index (BMI)

Classification	BMI category (kg/m^2)	Risk of developing health problems
Underweight	< 18.5	Increased
Normal weight	18.5–24.9	Least
Overweight	25.0–29.9	Increased
Obese class I	30.0–34.9	High
Obese class II	35.0–39.9	Very high
Obese class III	> 40.0	Extremely high

Source: Health Canada. *Canadian Guidelines for Body Weight Classification in Adults.* Ottawa: Minister of Public Works and Government Services Canada, 2003.

Most adults with a *high BMI* (overweight or obese) have a high percentage of body fat. Extra body fat is associated with an increased risk of health problems such as diabetes, heart disease, high blood pressure, gallbladder disease and some forms of cancer. A *low BMI* (underweight) is associated with health problems such as osteoporosis, undernutrition and eating disorders.

The higher your BMI falls outside the "normal weight" category, the higher your risk of developing weight-related health problems. It is important to note that sudden or considerable weight gains or weight losses may also indicate health risk, even if this occurs within the "normal weight" BMI category.

Excess fat around the waist and upper body (an "apple" body shape) is associated with greater health risk than fat located more in the hip and thigh area (a "pear" body shape). A waist measurement at or above 102 centimeters (40 inches) for men and 88 centimeters (35 inches) for women is associated with an increased risk of developing health problems such as diabetes, heart disease and high blood pressure. The cutoff points are approximate, so a waist circumference just below these values should also be taken seriously. In general, the higher the measurement above these cutoff points, the higher your risk of developing health problems. Even if your BMI is in the "normal weight" range, a high waist circumference indicates some health risk.

Staying Hydrated

Without a doubt, water is your best choice of fluids. Drinking water helps to regulate body temperature, shuttle nutrients to cells and muscles, shuttle waste products from the body, regulate metabolism and prevent hunger and increase cognition.

As a person who exercises regularly, water plays an important part in your fitness regime. The human body is made up of more than 70 percent water, so it's not surprising that dehydration can cause an impact in

 If you are obese, you may also be at risk for high blood pressure, liver disease, high cholesterol and type II diabetes. Diabetes is a permanent condition and occurs when the body doesn't produce enough insulin or when the cells in your body ignore the insulin. Your body needs insulin in order to use sugars. Foods that are easily converted into sugar, such as milk, bread, rice and fruit, give us the energy we require to live.

 The accumulation of excess weight is like the compounding of interest... when compounded on a daily basis, it can add up. And it is the difference between energy in and energy out that, when added up, can lead to excess weight gain. In other words, as Dr. Finegood says, "It's not what you do on an occasional basis, it's about what you do every day—how much energy you take in over what you expend—that makes a difference."

exercise performance with as little as 2 percent water loss. It doesn't take much to cause a 2 percent water loss: prolonged exercise, an illness such as the flu, hot weather or even a lack of drinking can cause dehydration.

Watch for the signs that indicate dehydration, including:

- an unexpected increase in heart rate
- increased perceived exertion (exercise feels harder than it should)
- small amounts of dark yellow urine
- thirst
- light-headedness and headaches
- muscle cramps

Lenny

Lenny is a 48-year-old nurse who became a regular walker after suffering a heart attack 5 years ago. Using a gradual and progressive walking program, he went from being a couch potato to a person who commutes 30 minutes on foot, to and from work.

A couple of months ago, Lenny decided to increase his walking time to prepare for a 6-mile (10-kilometer) charity walk/run event. In preparation for the event, he began to include a 2-hour walk on Saturday afternoons as part of his regular walking program. He loved the new challenge of the longer walks and the increased strength and endurance they provided. Unfortunately, he arrived home from these walks feeling fatigued, sluggish and incredibly hungry and would sleep on the couch for several hours before getting up for a late dinner. The next morning he would wake up with an incredible headache.

After enduring this pattern for more than a month, Lenny spoke with his family physician about his concerns, and she suggested that he meet with a dietitian. The dietitian analyzed Lenny's eating patterns and exercise habits and realized that he was not paying enough attention to staying hydrated and to eating before and after his long walks. After following the dietitian's hydration and pre- and post-fueling suggestions for a few weeks, Lenny is pleased that he no longer feels fatigued after his Saturday walks and that his headaches (likely caused by dehydration) are gone.

Your ultimate hydration goal is to never be thirsty again. Once thirst has set in, you are already dehydrated and can suffer the ill effects.

Commonly Asked Questions about Fluids

Q. *How much do I need to drink throughout the day?*

A. The following chart lists the amount of liquid you need to take in, depending on your age and body weight. Remember that fluids include water and all beverages and soups as well as things like popsicles and Jell-O. Limit the amount of tea and coffee you drink, to avoid dehydration. For example, if you are a 30-year-old female weighing 180 pounds (82 kilograms), convert 180 lb. x 0.45 kg per lb. = 81 kg. Multiply 81 kg x 40 mL per kg = 3,240 mL per day. So, you need to drink at least 3.2 liters (12 cups) of liquid per day.

Age	Basic fluid needs
16–30 years	40 mL per kg body weight per day
30–55 years	35 mL per kg body weight per day
55–75 years	30 mL per kg body weight per day
> 75 years	25 mL per kg body weight per day

Q. *If I'm exercising, when and how much should I drink?*

A. If you are active, aim for additional hydration. Use the following chart to guide you.

Time	Fluid Needs
Before exercise	1¼ to 2 cups (300 to 500 mL) an hour before activity
During exercise	3 to 4 large gulps every 15 minutes
After exercise	2 to 3 cups (500 to 750 mL) within an hour of activity

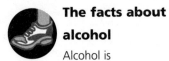

The facts about alcohol

Alcohol is dehydrating and has lots of calories, so it is not a good choice when you are exercising. In fact, alcohol has almost twice the number of calories per gram (7) as carbohydrates and proteins (4) do. Compare this with fat, which has 9 calories per gram. As well, alcohol delays the body's ability to recover and repair itself after exercise.

Q. *Should I drink sport drinks?*

A. Sport drinks contain water and carbohydrates in the form of simple sugars with added electrolytes like sodium and potassium. Sport drinks can be used if you are active longer than 1½ hours, since your body is likely to be depleted of electrolytes and muscle glycogen. Remember that if you're standing at the soda machine and think that choosing a sport drink is better for you than a cola, you're wrong. Both contain simple sugars and empty calories that, if consumed in excess, will be stored as fat. You can also make your own sport drink at home. Mix half juice with half water and add a pinch of salt!

Q. *Is it possible to drink too much?*

A. Yes. You might be surprised to learn that it *is* possible to drink too much water. Overhydration, also known as hyponatremia, can occur when you take in more water than your body is able to excrete, causing your sodium levels to be diluted. The first symptoms of overhydration include blurred vision, muscle cramps, twitching, rapid breathing, nausea and vomiting. If left untreated it can become extremely hazardous, even fatal.

Fourteen Tips for Healthy Eating and Drinking

It's a great idea to know your baseline before starting any exercise or healthy eating plan. Jennifer Gibson offers the following fourteen tips that can help you get started on a nutrition makeover for life. Remember to consult your family doctor and registered dietitian before undertaking a new diet.

1. *Keep track!* Keep track of everything you eat and drink over the next week, in a food journal. Write down the type of food or beverage and the amount. Take a look at what you're eating and why you're eating it. Use this information to prepare a menu plan that's right for your schedule.

2. *Buy a scale and weigh yourself on a regular basis.* Use a scale as a way to keep yourself on track. Track your weight loss to stay motivated. Don't get overly concerned about daily minor fluctuations; track your weight trend over time. This is especially important if you have a high-risk BMI.

3. *Become a planner.* Plan ahead for meals and snacks so you know exactly what you plan to eat. Do not go longer than 4 hours without eating.

4. *Cut your fat intake in half.* Have half as much margarine or butter on toast, vegetables and your muffin; half the mayonnaise on your sandwich, and half the oil in the pan when you sauté foods.

5. *Say not tonight, sweetie!* Limit the amount of sugary and fatty treats to two to three times per week *maximum*. Remember the 80/20 rule. Try to eat healthily 80 percent of the time.

6. *Make milk matter.* If you're not currently using skim milk, decrease the fat content in the milk you use. For example, if you currently use 2 percent, use only 1 percent. If you insist on whole milk, try 2 percent.

7. *Choose fruit.* Eat at least two servings of fresh fruit every day. Choose whatever type of fruit is in season.

8. *Become a "vegehead."* Include two servings of vegetables with lunch and dinner, for a total of at least four servings per day.

9. *Eat whole grains.* Choose one to two servings of foods made from whole grains with every meal.

10. *Make protein count.* Include good sources of protein at each meal, such as chicken, fish, legumes, peanut butter, cottage cheese, eggs, tofu or yogurt.

11. *Go meatless.* Eat at least one meatless lunch and dinner each week to reduce fat, increase fiber and get yourself into the habit of building meals around whole grains, beans and vegetables.

12. *Ditch the juice!* Instead of fruit juice for breakfast or a snack, drink water. Add a slice of lemon or lime for zest.

13. *Purge the processed.* Look through your cupboards for highly processed foods. Go fresh when you can. "Quick" preparation foods are usually high in salt and fat and low in nutrition.

14. *Turn off the tube!* Shut off the TV whenever you eat— that includes meals and snacks. Studies show that we automatically eat larger portions when we snack in front of the tube, and typically those foods are high in fat and sugar, which means excess calories.

Healthy meals in minutes

Meals that take less than 10 minutes to prepare! So simple, the ingredient list is the recipe!

Fruit Smoothie

1 cup (250 mL) fruit (fresh or frozen)

1 cup (250 mL) low-fat yogurt (any flavor)

2 cups (500 mL) vanilla soy milk or skim milk

Ice (optional)

Wash and cut the fruit. Combine all ingredients in a blender, blend on high for 3 minutes and serve.

Greek Omelet

1 to 2 eggs or ½ cup (125 mL) liquid egg
replacement, beaten

1 to 2 oz. (30 to 60 g) feta cheese

3 to 4 tbsp (45 to 60 mL) salsa or chopped tomato

Pinch of ground pepper

Combine eggs, cheese, salsa (or tomato) and pepper in a bowl. In a frying pan on medium heat, cook eggs for 3 to 5 minutes. (As the eggs cook, lift the edge of the omelet and tilt the pan, allowing any uncooked egg to run onto the hot surface.) Serve immediately.

Meatless Burger

1 soy burger

1 whole grain bun

Ketchup

Mustard

1 to 2 slices tomato

½ cup (125 mL) shredded lettuce

Toast the soy burger according to the directions on the package. Toast the bun, if you like. Slide the cooked burger onto the bun, then garnish with ketchup, mustard, tomato and lettuce. Season with salt and pepper.

Yogurt Parfait

6 oz. (170 g) plain or flavored low-fat yogurt

1 cup (250 mL) whole grain cereal or low-fat granola

1 cup (250 mL) berries (fresh or frozen)

or banana

Combine all ingredients in a bowl and serve.

Alison

Alison is a 35-year-old tax lawyer who couldn't believe her eyes when she tried to get into her favorite pair of walking shorts while packing for a hard-earned vacation. After stepping on her bathroom scale, it was clear she had gained 10 pounds (4.5 kilograms) in the previous 6 months. Between the long hours she had been putting in at the firm and her nonexistent exercise program, it was understandable that she was not at her ideal weight. In an effort to fit into her bikini, Alison immediately eliminated most of the carbohydrates from her diet and managed to lose 6 pounds (2.7 kilograms) in 2 weeks. Unfortunately, she found her diet virtually impossible to maintain while on holiday, and she quickly gained back the weight she had lost, plus an additional few pounds.

When Alison returned from her holiday, she asked a registered dietitian for help with her weight loss woes. After recording everything she ate over the course of 3 days and reviewing the details of her diet, Alison and her dietitian realized that she needed a more balanced approach to nutrition: more fruits, vegetables, protein and good fat, and fewer processed foods. As well, Alison was determined to find time in her day for regular exercise, both to help lose weight and to alleviate stress. She now packs a lunch for work and has started an afternoon walking group. At about 2:00 PM each day, she and a few lawyers from her firm get together for a brisk 30-minute walk. In less than 4 months, Alison has lost almost 10 pounds (4.5 kilograms). Besides being able to fit into her old clothes, she has more energy than she's had in several years.

Healthy Eating and Walking Go Hand in Hand

You've heard it said many times before that change takes time. This is true for every area of your life, including your diet. However, healthy living doesn't mean a life without fun. It's true that if you want to lose some extra weight you might have to forgo the beer, pizza and cream-filled doughnuts on a regular basis, but this doesn't mean you have to completely eliminate them from your diet. It's all about moderation.

It's a little-known secret that the psychological benefits of exercise can have a positive impact on your diet. It makes sense to think that the positive feelings you experience from regular exercise will spill over into other areas of your life. Once you feel healthier and better about yourself, it will become easier to make healthy choices in other areas. If you decide to make more nutritious food choices part of your new, active lifestyle, you'll quickly realize that the benefits of healthy eating far outweigh the negatives. After a nutritious meal you will begin to appreciate how much better you feel than when you devour a fast-food dinner. Soon you will want to feel good all the time, and once this happens the healthy choice will become the easy choice. And, as a person who exercises, you'll appreciate that the better the fuel you put in your tank, the better your body will perform.

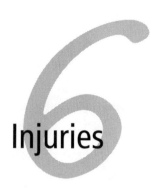

Injuries

TIME, PATIENCE AND CONSISTENCY: THESE ARE THE THREE
keys to success for any good exercise program. A walking program
is great for the body, mind and spirit, but there is a potential down-
side. Walking means extra stress is placed on the body, which can
sometimes lead to aches, pains and even injuries. Fortunately, most
walking-related injuries are avoidable if you understand how your
body works. If you do happen to get injured, there is valuable information in this chapter on what you need to do to get healthy and
return to your walking program.

How Your Body Will Change

Your body will undergo significant changes as you adapt to the physical demands of a regular walking program. To go from a sedentary
to an active lifestyle where you regularly walk for exercise, your body
must change, but remember that this will take time. Becoming fitter and staying injury free requires a good balance of work and rest.
Improved fitness actually occurs on rest days, when your body has
time to adapt to the hard work of your previous training session.

Without allowing yourself a sufficient recovery time, or rest, your body will not get stronger; it will just get more tired or, worse, sidelined by an injury.

Expecting change

Dr. Bryan Barootes describes how your body will change as you begin to exercise:

- Initially you will experience some muscle soreness/stiffness, as you are using muscles that you may not have exercised for many years. This soreness/stiffness should decrease as you continue with your program.
- You will notice improvements in the muscle tone in your legs and in your balance and flexibility. This will reduce your risk of falling.
- Your weight loss may be gradual; however, even 2 or 3 pounds (0.9 to 1.4 kilograms) will reduce the load on your joints and the resulting feelings of pain and stiffness.
- You will observe improved cardiac and respiratory fitness, which will improve your endurance and your ability to perform daily tasks.
- You may become more mentally alert, as exercise stimulates the brain.
- You will become more mobile and independent.
- If you have peripheral vascular disease, you will notice a reduction in leg pain. It has been proved that a structured fitness program is as effective as some medications.

Listening to your body

Each person is different. Therefore, what works for one does not necessarily work for the next. Essential to increasing your strength and endurance is the ability to listen to your body. This means being able to differentiate between an off day, when you lack motivation to get out the door for your walk, and feelings of extreme fatigue or aching muscles resulting from a previous workout session.

Not listening to what your body is telling you is one of the most common mistakes that leads to overuse injuries—chronic injuries resulting from overtraining. Vancouver sport physician Dr. Jim Bovard says that new exercisers are often quite goal oriented and enthusiastic and can easily persist with a walking program at the expense of developing overuse injuries.

Dr. Bovard stresses that regardless of the quality of the fitness program, each time a person starts exercising, he or she is an experiment of one. In other words, what works in general in a program will not apply 100 percent to the people using it. It is important to realize that experiencing pain when you walk is not supposed to happen. If one of your goals is to complete a specific 5- or 10-kilometer event, and you find that you need extra time to recover from an injury or just to build strength and endurance, you can always pick another event. Pushing through an injury will only make it worse. Remember, your walking program is intended to be part of a larger goal: making a healthy change in your lifestyle so that you can keep walking long after you reach the finish line of one particular event.

<table>
<tr>
<td>

Stay in tune with your body

Pay attention to any small aches or pains, and record them in your logbook. This will help you understand that it takes time for your body to build strength and stamina.

</td>
</tr>
</table>

Knowing when to rest and when to back off

If during one of your walk sessions you experience a pain that lasts until the next day, Dr. Bovard suggests that you take a few days off until it settles down. You can resume walking with less intensity than before and gradually build the intensity back to your previous level. If pain persists for more than 4 to 5 days, you need to see a health care professional with sport medicine expertise.

Bovard recommends that when you return to exercise following an injury, you should be pain free during day-to-day activities such as walking up stairs, and you should have full range of motion and strength in the injured area. Once you've reached this point, use a gradual and progressive approach to return to a regular walking program. If you do too much too soon, you will end up back where you were before you started your recovery process.

Commonly Asked Questions about Injury

Q. *Will I feel stiff and sore?*

A. Yes. Even though the programs in this book are designed to be gradual and progressive, it is normal for your body to feel a little stiff and sore from time to time throughout your training program. After all, it will take time for your muscles, tendons and ligaments to respond to the increased demands of a regular exercise program. To build strength and endurance, you need to progressively overload the muscles to stimulate them and then allow them time to recover. The overloading causes small tears in the muscle fibers, which you notice when you feel sore or stiff 24 to 48 hours after an exercise session. When resting, the muscles repair themselves and become stronger than before.

Q. *Is the mantra "no pain, no gain" true for all exercise programs?*
A. Absolutely not. However, a certain degree of stiffness, soreness and tiredness is unavoidable when you first begin exercising. The gradual approach of the programs in this book minimizes the likelihood of injury. Remember, the goal is for you to adopt an active lifestyle where you walk regularly for fitness, not to get to the start line of your chosen event by taking shortcuts, skipping workout sessions or jumping ahead in your walking program.

Q. *What does it mean to "pace" yourself?*
A. Pacing is the process of establishing a walking speed that you can maintain throughout the duration of your walk. Finding a pace that works for you can be challenging. In the beginning, it's better to go a little slower than you would like than too fast. This way, you will complete your walk feeling you could have walked much farther. The last thing you want to do is to be so tired at the end of your walk that it takes days to recover, forcing you to skip future workouts or, worse, become sick or injured. A good way to tell if you're walking at a good pace is to give yourself the talk test (see chapter 2).

Q. *Why is it not a good idea to walk on consecutive days?*
A. Fatigue, and sometimes soreness, often peaks

during the 48 hours after a workout session. If you're still tired or your muscles are sore the next time you're scheduled to walk, don't hesitate to take an extra rest day. If you can remain somewhat flexible as to when you walk, it will reduce your chances of overuse injuries.

Q. *How can keeping a logbook help to prevent injuries?*
A. By keeping a regular written account of your training sessions, you can see the big picture and the patterns that emerge over time. These records enable you to analyze and monitor your progress. As well, a logbook helps you to closely monitor your aches and pains or feelings of fatigue; later, if needed, it acts as a resource for understanding injuries or illness.

Q. *I'm overweight. Are there any injuries that will be more common for me?*
A. Dr. Barootes says that individuals who are overweight are more prone to dehydration and heat-related illness, so fluid replacement is essential. Refer to chapter 5 for information on hydration.

Q. *As a diabetic with neuropathy, am I predisposed to specific injuries?*
A. Neuropathy is a disease of the nerves that has many causes, including diabetes. Symptoms range from a tingling sensation or numbness in the toes and fingers to paralysis. Dr. Barootes suggests that if you have diabetes or neuropathy (from any cause), you are at greater risk of foot-related problems and *must* inspect your feet daily and after exercise. Look for cuts, scratches, abrasions

and irritations from your shoes and socks. Check the top and bottom of your feet as well as between your toes. If you are diabetic, check your sugars before and after exercise and carry appropriate glucose replacement if you are hypoglycemic. As well, only use NSAIDS (non-steroid anti-inflammatory drugs such as Advil, ibuprofen and Aleve, used to manage arthritis or joint pain) with your doctor's permission, as you may be very sensitive to the effects these drugs have on your kidney functioning. Finally, be sure to get the green light from your family doctor before starting your walking program.

Assessing Your Aches and Pains

As you progress through your walking program, a few minor aches and pains are unavoidable. You are the best judge of how you feel, so learning how to read your level

Ginny

Ginny is a 72-year-old hairdresser who owns a small hair salon in Ann Arbor, Michigan. As a child growing up in Phoenix, Arizona, and then as a college student at Arizona State University, Ginny was an avid walker. Even during the extraordinarily hot summers, she loved nothing more than meeting her girlfriends for their 5:00 AM speed-walking session.

After meeting her husband, Hank, and moving to Michigan, Ginny continued to speed walk regularly. She had had few walking-related injuries, until she tore her hamstring muscle in a bad fall on a patch of ice. Having been an athlete for most of her life, it was difficult for Ginny to take time off from walking, and she became withdrawn and moody.

In an effort to cheer up his wife, Hank suggested a 2-week vacation in her home state. Ginny jumped at the thought of the Arizona sun; it motivated her and boosted her mood. As a way of easing herself back into speed walking, she began with short walks at an easy pace. By the end of the 2 weeks she was able to walk for 30 minutes without pain. Ginny was thrilled with her recovery and returned to Michigan ready to ease herself into speed walking, though a little more carefully on the ice.

If you're having repeated problems with your feet, knees or hips, see a sport medicine podiatrist. This specialist will look at your body's alignment and may suggest custom-made orthotics to correct any biomechanical problems.

of pain and to trust your judgment is essential to reducing your chances of injury or illness.

Use an injury-awareness scale

An injury-awareness scale can help you prevent a minor ache from becoming a serious issue. In your mind, create an imaginary 10-point scale on which "1" equals very little pain and "10" represents an extremely high level of pain. Ideally, your level of pain should be at around 1 or 2. If it is any higher than 4, you have returned to activity too soon and need to extend your recovery period. It's important to be honest and to closely monitor your pain. If the pain persists for longer than a few days and if it gets higher than 5 or so, you need to talk to a sport medicine physician for guidance in deciding on the appropriate recovery time. If you return to your walking program too soon, you often risk further injury.

Take a look at your technique

If you're having problems with your back or hips, have a friend or walking partner look at your walking technique. If you want to increase your speed, you may naturally be tempted to lengthen your stride. Be careful that you're not overextending your leg in an effort to reach too far forward. Instead of making you go faster, this extra-long stride leads to a clumsy gait because your foot strikes the ground with added force, causing your feet and shins unnecessary stress and pain.

Keep in mind that when you walk, your main power source comes from pushing with the back leg and foot. If you want to walk faster, use short, quick steps. Focus on rolling your foot forward from heel to toe to get a strong push off. Your stride will lengthen naturally when your foot efficiently pushes off from the ground, which will in turn improve your pace.

Common Injuries

Dr. Barootes says that, initially, the most common complaints from new exercisers are muscle soreness, blisters and calluses, which indicate either a level of walking that is too intense or improper footwear or socks. As walkers progress into a walking program, the more serious injuries are usually related to the feet, shins, knees and back and are usually the result of overuse, or doing too much too soon.

Small aches and pains

With any kind of exercise program, you are bound to feel a few minor aches and pains. On the surface they may be small concerns in comparison with an injury, but if left untreated, they can interrupt your training schedule and leave you feeling frustrated and discouraged. By understanding the signs, symptoms and treatment of these minor aches and pains you should be able to easily treat yourself and be back on the road in no time. If, however, problems persist, please seek medical attention from your health care provider.

Chafing

Chafing often occurs on the inner thighs, groin area, armpits and nipples as a result of sweating and of friction from body parts rubbing together or from

Stay relaxed
Try to keep your shoulders and arms loose, especially when you begin to feel fatigued. Swing your arms and press the tips of your thumbs against the tips of another finger, as if you are about to snap your fingers. The concentrated pressure point helps to relax the shoulders and upper body.

When walking, each foot strikes the ground about eight hundred times per kilometer. The arms swing in rhythm with the feet. That's a lot of body parts rubbing against each other, hundreds of times every outing. The clothing you wear, especially its seams and texture, can get caught in between these passing limbs, setting up a perfect environment for chafing and blisters. Minimize this effect by choosing synthetic clothing with flat seams and applying Vaseline or skin lubricant where friction commonly occurs, such as between your thighs and under your arms.

clothing. A chafed area is usually red, raw and possibly bleeding. You will need to wash and clean the area to avoid infection and cover it with a sterile, nonstick pad that will allow it to breathe until it is healed. To prevent chafing, drink plenty of water before, during and after walking. Staying hydrated will help preclude the rubbing and allow your body to perspire naturally. When you stop perspiring, your sweat forms salt crystals on your body, which increases friction. It's also a good idea to wear breathable clothing. See Avoiding Common Injuries later in this chapter for more information on quick-drying clothes.

Blisters

Blisters are localized accumulations of fluid between layers of skin. They're usually caused by friction on the skin due to poorly fitting shoes, improper taping and/or overuse. A "hot spot" (a warm, reddened area) is the precursor to a blister. Continued friction and irritation can lead to the formation of a serum-filled (clear fluid) blister or, less commonly, a blood-filled blister. Some of the signs that a blister may soon form are swelling, redness and pain. If you do have a blister, treat it by washing and cleaning the area thoroughly with soapy water. Next, apply alcohol over the area, and carefully poke a sterile needle into the blister. Gently remove the fluid using a sterile gauze pad, and finally cover the blister with Second Skin or a sterile, nonstick pad and secure it with medical tape. Vaseline or skin lubricant should be applied liberally over the area to reduce any further friction from your sock and shoe. To avoid blisters, try to keep your feet as dry as possible and free from ill-fitting sock seams. If the seams on your socks do cause rubbing, try wearing your socks inside out.

Athlete's foot

Athlete's foot (*Tinea pedis*) is a fungal infection that commonly affects the feet but can also occur on the head, body, skin and nails. Common symptoms include itchy feet; an initial rash; dry, scaly skin, and cracks in the skin between the toes. If left untreated, the fungus progresses to large patches of flaky skin. To treat athlete's foot, ask your pharmacist to suggest a topical cream. When applying the antifungal cream, it's important to keep the area as dry as possible. To prevent athlete's foot from occurring in the first place, remove damp shoes and socks as soon as possible, clean your shower regularly, and when using community showers make sure you wear flip-flops or other plastic sandals.

Muscle cramps

Muscle cramps are painful contractions or spasms of a muscle usually caused by fatigue, water loss or inadequate stretching and conditioning. They most often occur when the muscle is hit, overstretched or used with too much force. The common signs include sudden, sharp and severe pain, usually when you are walking but sometimes after a long walk. The cramped area may feel like a hard knot, with an involuntary contraction of the muscle. To treat muscle cramps, apply ice for 10 to 15 minutes to relax the muscle and reduce the pain. Gentle stretching can be effective. Be sure to take in enough fluids to prevent or help alleviate cramping, as cramps can be one of the first signs of heat illness. If the cramping muscle doesn't respond to any of these suggestions or to a massage, you should assume that some tissue may be damaged. Consult your family doctor for a proper diagnosis. To prevent cramping, ease into your walk sessions and be sure to stay properly hydrated.

Abdominal stitches

A "stitch" is a common abdominal pain that's often brought about by a muscle spasm of the diaphragm or by eating too much and too close to walking. The muscle spasms usually arise because not enough oxygen is getting to the muscle, either because of poor conditioning, improper breathing techniques and/or an insufficient supply of blood to the diaphragm. Other reasons for stitches include constipation, intestinal gas, a distended spleen or weak abdominal muscles. Some of the symptoms include a sharp pain on either side of the diaphragm, usually below the rib cage. To treat a stitch in your side, relax the spasm area by changing your walking stride length or decreasing your pace. Using your hand, apply pressure over the area, or stop walking completely until the pain subsides. If the pain persists, try raising the arm of the affected side over your head and stretch. You can continue your walking session once the stitch is gone.

Avoiding Common Injuries

1. *Wear synthetic clothing.* For every 2,000 steps you take, you burn about 500 calories, which causes your body

to heat up. As your core temperature increases, your body begins to perspire in order to cool itself. Understandably, the more you perspire, the greater the moisture you create, making your clothes wet and uncomfortable. A wet garment that slightly rubs a sensitive area of the body will increase friction and potentially cause an abrasion or a blister. Cotton can absorb up to seven times its weight in water, whereas the new synthetic nylons and polyesters will wick moisture away from the skin and through the garment, allowing it to dissipate into the air. With this dry garment next to your skin, you cut down on abrasion and increase comfort.

2. *Lubricate and protect problem areas.* For those who walk significant distances, lubricants such as Vaseline and special antifriction roll-ons (sold at athletic stores) as well as gel-like blister pads (for example, Second Skin) can help manage problem areas between the thighs and around the underarms, nipples and bra lines. Don't forget duct tape: in problem areas, it sticks better than anything else in damp conditions and is very slick and nonabrasive on the skin.

3. *Dress for the weather.* Managing the cold and the rain is a challenge. The key is to stay dry from the inside out, as well as from the outside in. Phil Moore, a sportswear specialist, suggests that you *always* wear a synthetic moisture-wicking layer right against your skin. There are lots of materials with proprietary names like CoolMax and DryFit. Keeping the clothing against your skin dry is essential for a comfortable walk. Add warm layers such as fleece or wool

and/or a jacket, if necessary. If it's raining, the outer layer of clothing should be a water-resistant, breathable garment. Avoid rain jackets that are fully waterproof but don't breathe. They are no better than wearing a garbage bag with a couple of arm holes cut out! In the end, clothing should be comfortable and manage moisture well.

Plantar fasciitis

Plantar fasciitis is a stretching or inflammation of the tissue that runs along the sole of your foot. The plantar fascia is a collection of connective tissue originating at the bottom of the heel and progressing towards the ball of the foot. This area helps to maintain the arch and acts as an impact absorber. Plantar fasciitis is usually a chronic condition, brought on by pronated (or flat) feet, high arches, wearing shoes with inadequate arch support, and weak or inflexible muscles in the lower leg and foot. Signs and symptoms include pain along the arch or near the bottom of the heel, inability to push off with the foot or point the foot down, pain and an inability to walk without limping, especially in the morning or after prolonged periods of sitting. There may also be lumps on the underside of the foot, especially near the heel. To treat plantar fasciitis, rest and apply ice to reduce the inflammation and help with pain control. Strengthen your foot muscles by doing towel curls or picking up objects with your toes. If the pain persists, you may need your family doctor to prescribe anti-inflammatory medication or other treatments.

Sprained ankle

A sprained ankle occurs when your foot twists, rolls or turns beyond your normal range of motion, causing the ligaments that hold the ankle bones and joint in position to stretch beyond their normal length. If the force is too strong, the ligaments can tear. Common symptoms of a sprained ankle include pain and difficulty standing on and stabilizing the injured foot. How much pain and how unstable you are depend on how much the ligament has been stretched or torn. To treat a sprained ankle, keep your ankle elevated above your heart level as much as possible for the first 48 hours.

Steve

Steve is an adrenaline junkie. He's 44 years old, but when he races his motorbike at the weekend motocross races, you would think he was closer to 25. Unfortunately, he had a bad crash last season that resulted in a broken collarbone and two broken legs. It took three months before he was able to get out of bed without help.

After his accident, Steve gained a little weight and his fitness declined. But the biggest concern was his mood—whereas he had previously been full of life, with energy for everyone and everything, he had become withdrawn, rarely returned his friends' phone messages and spent his time watching television.

One day, after months of watching Steve sit alone in his apartment, his brother, Pete, went to the apartment and forced Steve to get outside for a short walk around the block. Pete returned the next day, and every day after that. At first, Steve had to use a cane to support himself, but within a few weeks he was ready to try walking without it. Although he wasn't quite ready for this step and had to lean on his brother's shoulder for the walk home, the point is he tried.

The walks were not a magic pill that returned Steve to his former self, but they were the first steps towards his recovery. He soon agreed to regular physiotherapy treatment and continued a gradual and progressive walking program. While Steve would have preferred to be on the track riding his motorbike, he enjoyed being outside and was able to make walking a big part of his rehabilitation program.

Treat yourself to a massage

A massage works wonders for the legs, back and your general well-being. If your partner isn't willing, splurge on a therapeutic massage after you've stayed committed to your program and put some good weeks behind you.

Rest the injured leg, and apply ice for 20 to 30 minutes, three to four times a day to decrease the swelling, pain and dysfunction. Apply pressure to the injured area using bandages or ice-wraps to immobilize and support the injured ankle. The healing process takes anywhere from 4 to 6 weeks, but make an appointment with your family doctor for a complete diagnosis and treatment guidelines.

Sore knees

The heavier you are, the more stress there will be on your knee joints. This increased stress often leads to sore knees after walking. To avoid injury, start with shorter walking segments, as suggested by Dr. Barootes in chapter 2. Then gradually increase your walking time and pace. Using ice after exercise may also help reduce swelling and stiffness (see Treating Common Injuries at Home at the end of this chapter). As well, fitness consultant Diana Rochon recommends focusing on keeping your knees soft (slightly bent) when you walk and extending your leg through your hip by using your gluteus (buttocks) muscles to propel you forward. Remember, if knee pain or swelling worsens or persists, see your family doctor to ensure that you are not causing problems to your joints.

Back pain

Fitness consultant Diana Rochon says, "Low-back stiffness is common for new walkers. If you haven't been very active, chances are that your overall posture and the mobility of your lower back could be better." To

Walking for Fitness

combat lower-back pain, concentrate on stretching after each walk as well as incorporating a hamstring and low-back stretch prior to your walk. Focus on your walking posture for 30 seconds at a time during your walk. Easy posture cues to focus on include keeping your eyes focused on the horizon, making sure your breastbone is gently tilted up to the sky and ensuring that your hips are up and forward (think of your hip bones as headlights and "shine" them straight ahead!). To avoid mental overload, focus on just one of these posture cues at a time. Improving your posture will decrease the strain on your lower back. If the stiffness in your lower back continues or worsens (pain), see your doctor or physiotherapist for additional help.

Neck and shoulders

Although you don't walk on your neck or shoulders, Rochon says that it's common for people to hunch their shoulders, clench their fists and generally hold tension in the upper part of their body while walking. The tightness in the upper body will only make your walking more tedious and less pleasant. Try to focus on maintaining a relaxed upper body during your walks: look at your reflection in a store window or have your walking partner check that your neck and shoulders are dropped down away from your ears.

Avoiding More Serious Injuries

1. *Progress slowly.* If you review the programs in this book, you will see that the progressions are slow and deliberate. It is important *not* to increase your

activity level by more than 10 percent a week. The leading cause of injuries for new exercisers is walking too far before they're ready. Remember that your focus is on the time spent in your workout, *not* the distance that you cover.

2. *Choose your training surface wisely.* Asphalt is the surface on which most walkers log the most miles. Although it is not the softest surface, asphalt is a little easier on your joints than concrete. Try to walk on the most level part of the road or pathway, since cambered roads will lead to imbalance and possible injury. Be alert for hard-to-see bumps, holes, sprinklers and tree roots when walking on grass and dirt trails.

Marlene

Marlene is a 65-year-old retired communication studies professor. She's been walking for pleasure for as long as she can remember. Marlene grew up on a farm in Ontario and recalls the joy of walking in the forest with her father, who taught her the names of the local trees, plants and birds. She also has fond memories of walking with her sister to play at the creek. From age 6, Marlene enjoyed the 2-mile (3-kilometer) walk to and from their one-room country schoolhouse, singing as she went, watching the birds and animals and looking for wild strawberries or apples. In retrospect, Marlene says, "I've always associated walking with pleasure, with time to relate to nature and to just let my mind float freely. My body and psyche miss walking a lot if I can't do it."

Since retirement, Marlene usually walks 6 days a week, for an average of 45 minutes at a fairly brisk pace, though she sometimes walks at a moderate pace if she's with friends. When she walks more slowly than usual, she will often carry small weights to get a more satisfying workout. Marlene walks more these days than she did in the past when she also did other physical activities such as swimming, using a gym or kayaking. However, she recently bought a new mountain bike, which she thoroughly enjoys and which competes a bit with walking! Marlene's health is excellent. At her annual checkup, her doctor said that she is probably the healthiest 65-year-old he will see this year.

3. *Don't walk with pain.* If something hurts, listen to your body. An ache is a low-level discomfort associated with exercising, while pain is a sharp discomfort whose source can be pinpointed. Pain is a warning sign that should not be ignored. In the beginning, there will always be a few aches and pains that come with starting a new activity. However, they should dissipate within 24 to 48 hours. If they don't, or if the pain intensifies, seek professional assistance. Early identification and treatment of an injury will result in minimal interruptions to your training schedule.

4. *Promptly treat injuries.* Muscle pulls, joint sprains or other injuries should be promptly treated using the RICE principles outlined below.

5. *Know when to "pack it in."* Some days, you just shouldn't exercise. If you've got the flu or a bad chest cold, take a couple of days off. Likewise, trying to exercise through an injury may result in the problem getting worse. What may have taken a few rest days to recover from ends up hobbling you for weeks. Better to take off an extra day or two or three, even if you think the pain isn't serious.

Treating Common Injuries at Home

RICE is the acronym for rest, ice, compression and elevation. It is a common and effective procedure used for treating injuries.

Rest is important to avoid an injury from getting worse. It doesn't mean you need to stop all activity; in most cases, in fact, complete rest is rarely recommended.

Stimulating blood flow to the injured soft tissue is necessary for healing. Speak with your sport medicine practitioner for suggestions on how best to strengthen the muscles around the injured area.

Ice is an effective way to minimize swelling, decrease pain from an injury and improve recovery time. Apply ice as quickly as possible, and do so for 20 minutes at a time. Leave about an hour between intervals, and be sure to place a thin wet cloth between the bag of ice and your skin.

Compression can be done using an elastic wrap like a tensor bandage to prevent swelling, reduce pain and minimize bruising. Compression should be firm but not tight, and the bandage should be left on for no more than 3 hours. It should never be left on overnight.

Elevation means raising the injured area above the heart to minimize pooling of blood and reduce swelling of the injured area.

This chapter should help you avoid injury, but if you find yourself unable to continue with your walking program, it doesn't necessarily mean that you will have to stop exercising altogether until you are completely healed. If your doctor doesn't object, you could try other activities to keep you active while you're injured, such as swimming or cycling. Besides keeping you active, new activities add variety and will provide you with all of the physical and mental benefits of your walking program. If you're careful and follow your doctor's instructions, you should be back walking in no time.

Walking for Fitness

Including the Family and Friends

FAMILIES WHO PLAY TOGETHER, HAVE FUN TOGETHER! Besides being a way to clear your mind, improve your health and get fit, walking is a great way to connect with loved ones. After all, catching up on the details of daily life is easier and more enjoyable during a walk to school or home from work than it is while driving in rush-hour traffic. As well, older children, and even some adults, find it's easier to share personal matters while walking, because there isn't the added anxiety of direct eye contact.

Unfortunately, in today's fast-paced society of cell phones, computers and fast-food outlets at every street corner, it isn't easy to become an active family. Making the healthy choice in terms of nutrition, exercise and lifestyle is the difficult choice, but it's a lifelong pursuit that is certain to bring huge rewards for you and your family. It will take time to organize, adapt and change old patterns, but this chapter provides you with all of the guidance and advice you'll need to get your family moving towards a healthier lifestyle.

i Most families have a calendar posted above the telephone or on the refrigerator door where they note upcoming events. On the same calendar, write down the details of your walking program such as time, duration and location of each of your walks. Writing down your fitness plan reconfirms your commitment and helps to keep your family in the loop. If your family knows that, for example, you walk every Monday after work, it helps them to be supportive. Posting your walk sessions will also minimize potential stress or conflict and, in turn, increase the likelihood of your meeting your walking goals.

Healthy Families Make a Healthy Society

When it comes to exercise and good nutrition, too many of us are on autopilot. Most of us understand the importance of exercise and healthy eating, yet we continue to ignore the staggering effects of our sedentary ways. We tell ourselves that we are too busy with our career, family and other demands to work out and plan proper meals. The problem is that this sedentary lifestyle is having hazardous effects on our health and the health of our children. Recent statistics indicate that close to half of all North American adults are overweight or obese.

A healthy lifestyle starts with parents. Most parents know that modeling good behavior is key, and exercise is no exception. If you can organize and motivate yourself to become a person who walks regularly, with a little encouragement your family won't be far behind. This isn't to say that carving out time is easy for any busy mom or dad, but with a little planning it can be done.

Walking during and after pregnancy

Pregnancy might seem an odd time to start a fitness program, but mom and baby can benefit from a gradual and progressive walking program. In fact, most health care providers agree that, if there are no complications with a pregnancy, maintaining a regular exercise program throughout pregnancy can help to keep your muscles and heart strong. Dr. Liz Joy, a Salt Lake City sport medicine physician, says, "I encourage all of my pregnant patients, even the previously sedentary ones, to stay active. A regular walking program is ideal for pregnant women who have been inactive in the past, are at risk for gestational diabetes or want to take a break from the high impact of running." Joy feels strongly that mom and baby can benefit from a gradual and progressive walking program.

If you're an expecting mom who wants to start or continue with a regular walking program, consider the following tips:

- Even if you were active prior to becoming pregnant, it's important to speak with your health care provider about your pregnancy fitness plans.
- Maintain a moderate exercise program throughout your pregnancy. This approach is better for you than infrequent but rigorous exercise sessions.
- Focus on being healthy. This is not the time to be drastically improving your fitness level.
- As your pregnancy progresses, you will likely find that you have to work harder than you were accustomed to in the earlier stages of pregnancy. If this is the case, ease back and modify your program to better meet your current fitness needs.
- Be sure to eat a good meal or snack 2 to 3 hours before exercising, and stay hydrated on your walks by always carrying a water bottle.
- Remember, you want to feel invigorated after your walk, not exhausted. Pregnancy is tiring enough without looking for ways to add stress.
- You'll notice that as you get farther into your pregnancy your center of gravity will change due to your larger frame, so be extra careful when you're walking.

Reasons to stay fit while pregnant

According to the book *Fit to Deliver: An Innovative Prenatal and Postpartum Fitness Program,* by Karen Nordahl and others, maintaining a regular exercise program, such as walking, throughout your pregnancy will help to improve your:

- body image
- circulation
- digestion
- endurance
- mood
- postpartum recovery
- self-esteem
- sense of well-being
- strength

Walking during pregnancy will reduce:

- backaches
- constipation
- leg cramps
- muscle swelling

- Pay close attention to your body. If it hurts, or if you feel dizzy, nauseous or uncomfortable, stop. If these feelings persist, be sure to check with your health care provider.

Walking after the baby arrives

After the baby arrives, most women can resume some light walking as soon as they feel ready, but it's important that you check with your health care provider for direction on your post-pregnancy walking plans. Most physicians recommend that women don't physically exert themselves until about 2 weeks after a vaginal birth and 6 to 8 weeks after a cesarean delivery. Each delivery is different, so be sure to check with your physician about any concerns that might prevent you from starting up a daily walking routine.

Walking with your baby

Walking with your baby is a great way to get out of the house and back on track with your own fitness goals. Keep in mind that it's never too early to introduce your baby to the joys of exercise and the outdoors. Walking is a great way to connect with your child even as a newborn! And just think: walking with your baby ensures that some of his or her first memories will be that exercising is fun and enjoyable.

A baby stroller can be a great way to walk with your child. Keep these tips in mind when using a stroller:

- When your child is just a newborn, avoid rough terrain. The bumps and vibrations from dirt and rock trails can be hard on a baby. Stick with leisurely walks on city sidewalks and quiet streets.

- When the baby has developed some neck strength, which is usually around 6 months, it should be okay to take short walks on rougher terrain.

- When walking with the stroller, try to avoid leaning forward into the stroller or backward, as this will encourage poor posture. Instead, focus on good walking posture (see chapter 3).

- Plan ahead as to how you will feed your baby. If you're a dad, or a mom who isn't nursing or who is not comfortable nursing in public, be sure to take a baby bottle in case your little one gets hungry.

- It's hard work to push a stroller, so make sure you carry extra water and a snack for yourself.

 Overcome child care anxieties
Search out your local gym or community center where child care is provided for a reasonable price. It takes a bit of organizing, but it can be a great way to get in your walking session and for your child to have time with other kids.

Madeline

Madeline is a 38-year-old elementary school teacher who loves to mountain bike, river kayak and snowshoe. When she's not heading for the mountains or the nearest river she's usually out on the playground coaching one of her school's many sports teams. A few months ago, Madeline and her partner, Gloria, were thrilled to receive the news that after 3 years of exhaustive efforts, Madeline was pregnant.

Madeline had already had two earlier miscarriages, so she wanted to be extra careful this time. She also wanted to continue being active, but she worried that her athletic lifestyle might jeopardize her chances of carrying the baby to term. Understanding that sports and the outdoors are a big part of Madeline's life, her doctor suggested that replacing Madeline's regular activities with a walking program might be the best way to stay fit.

At first, Madeline found walking to be a little boring. Then she started to walk in the trails near her work. She found the trails quiet and peaceful. Soon her walks became the favorite part of her day—they were a time to meditate and prepare herself for becoming a mother. Also, Gloria, who isn't very athletic, was pleased to be able to do an outdoor activity with Madeline.

The first baby gift they've received is a sturdy stroller that is designed for the trails. The two women are excited for the baby to arrive so that she, or he, can join them on their trail-walking adventures.

Encouraging Activity in Children

Just like adults, children receive huge benefits from an active lifestyle. Effective weight management, increased self-confidence and a healthy body are just a few of the many positives of an active childhood. As well, fit kids are known to be healthier, have better concentration skills and often grow up to be active adults. But what's surprising is that kids today are some of the least healthy people in our society. In North America and other parts of the world, children are fatter and less fit and have more health problems than ever before. The *International Journal of Pediatric Obesity* reports that almost half of North and South American children will be overweight by 2010.

Pediatrician Dr. Trent Smith says the strongest contributing factors to childhood obesity include:

- more screen-based activities, such as television, the Internet and video games, that are associated with low energy expenditure
- car-based transportation that has replaced walking and cycling
- increased automation, including TV remote controls, automated lawn watering and leaf blowers, which has contributed to a less vigorous lifestyle
- busier lives and an increased concern for safety, which makes parents less willing to permit free, spontaneous, unstructured active play among children and youth
- increased overall calorie consumption, with a dramatic increase in portion size and calorie contribution from "low-quality" foods such as fast food, soft

drinks and junk food. Studies show that children engaged in passive activities tend to eat more high-fat and high-calorie snack foods and, due to the distraction of their activity, often ignore internal signs that they are full and should stop eating.

Making fitness a family affair

Establishing fitness goals for your child can be difficult. Instead of thinking of exercise in terms of a single chunk of time, Dr. Smith suggests that parents encourage children to be active whenever possible; many small bouts of exercise done frequently throughout the day are often easier and more enjoyable for children and have the same health benefits as one large chunk of time. Smith suggests that older children and youth should strive to exercise for at least 90 minutes per day, at least 30 minutes of which should be vigorous (of sufficient intensity to increase the breathing rate and make the person warm).

Parental modeling is paramount. After a long workday, most parents are hard pressed to find enough time to prepare dinner for the family and help children with homework, never mind fitting in a game of catch in the backyard. Dr. Smith believes that it's a good idea for parents to make a conscious effort to walk, bicycle, rollerblade or skate to and from places, particularly in everyday commutes. Going for a family walk after dinner or walking together to school or on errands is important and can dramatically improve fitness and body shape. He also says that by and large there are few medical contraindications to becoming active, even for

 Limit "recreational" screen time to less than 90 minutes per day, and replace the time spent in front of the screen with time spent being physically active.

morbidly obese children or youth. For best success, reread chapter 2. Remember to start slowly, be sure the starting level of activity is appropriate and provide early, positive feedback. These three steps can do a world of good for establishing lifelong habits.

If you want to motivate your child to become more active, consider the following suggestions:

- *Encourage choice:* Allow your child to have a choice in the activity. Being inactive should not be an option, but the type of activity, within the financial and time constraints of a given family, should be the child's choice. Recognize that what your child views as fun this week may change next week or next month. Try to be flexible and accept that change and variety are good.

WALKER PROFILE

Clint

Clint is a 60-year-old retired marine officer. Several years ago, he and his wife moved into a condominium in Florida in a community with two pools, a tennis court and an area for shuffleboard. Although Clint had previously stayed fit for work, he put on about 20 pounds (9 kilograms) and became largely inactive once he retired.

After a few weeks in Florida, Clint met his neighbor, Bob. Most mornings, Bob walked for over an hour and then finished his walk with a cool dip in one of the pools. Clint was amazed by Bob's motivation, and he worked up the courage to ask Bob if he could join him on one of his walks. The two men started walking together and now, 4 years later, they still walk three mornings a week.

Clint hasn't lost all of his extra weight, but he feels great and loves having more energy. The best part about Clint's new walking routine, though, is the great friend he has found in his walking partner. He and Bob have shared many stories during their walks, from their shared passion for the Chicago Cubs to the birth of their grandchildren. Walking has definitely added to Clint's life in more ways than he could ever have imagined.

- *Explore nature:* Enjoy the fun and excitement of being outdoors by heading to your local park or green space with your children. Take along a guidebook that explains the birds, trees and flowers.

- *Learn to use a map:* Teach your child how to use a map. Find an easy-to-read city or park map and have your child use the map to find a destination of his or her choice. Or have your child draw his or her own map of your neighborhood, adding more details after each walk.

- *Search for a treasure:* If your child is a little older, teach him or her how to use a compass. Hide a treasure and write down the longitudinal and latitudinal directions on a piece of paper, then have your child search for the prize using the compass.

- *Plan a picnic:* Pack a lunch and walk to your destination. It's a great way to enjoy the outdoors, get some exercise and spend time with your child.

 Motivate your child to become more active

1. Set and enforce limits on the time spent in front of the television or computer.
2. Encourage your child to have a choice in the activity.
3. Explore nature in your local parks.
4. Try exploring the outdoors by learning to use a compass.
5. Use a map to find destinations your child is interested in.
6. Pack a lunch and walk to your destination.

An exercise plan for overweight children

If you have a child who is sedentary or overweight and you want him or her to make changes, try to keep in mind that change can be difficult for kids. Dr. Smith says that when he counsels overweight children, he tries to remind them that they are embarking on a lifelong plan for health and not a 2-month exercise program, so they don't have to change everything at once. However, obese children should be examined by a family doctor to rule out the chances of any "medical" cause for the weight problem.

Once your child has received the okay from a

Walking when you don't feel like it

There are bound to be days when you just don't feel like doing your walk, but trust me, you'll feel worse if you don't go. Be strong. Be committed. *Find a friend* for support. You don't want to see a blank spot in your walking diary. Nine times out of ten, if you make yourself lace up your shoes and head out the door, you'll be glad you did.

doctor to begin an exercise program, he or she needs to know that it will take time to get used to being active. In the early stages of a fitness program, it's common for heavy kids to complain that they are short of breath. This is likely a reflection of the increased work they do at any given speed (moving the extra mass), and in larger kids this reflects limitations in the movement of the chest wall due to excess fat. For this reason, it's essential that kids start out at a level that's appropriate for their fitness level. For guidelines on finding a suitable exercise pace, see chapter 2.

If you have older kids, try to expose them to as many different activities as possible. Just because certain activities are not of interest to you doesn't mean that will be the case for your son or daughter. As one physical education teacher points out, "The skateboarders at our school are one of the fittest groups in the school!"

Include the entire family

Regardless of age, walking is an ideal family activity that you can enjoy with loved ones of all ages. Consider inviting older parents, grandparents and great aunts and uncles the next time you're planning an outing. Depending on the level of fitness and interest, you might want to choose activities that are close to home and include benches or rest areas. Botanical gardens, farmers' markets, bird sanctuaries, museums and galleries are just a few examples of places you can explore with the entire family.

The Benefits of Walking Partners

One of the most successful motivators for keeping you on track with a regular fitness program is a good exercise partner. By making a commitment to regularly meet someone for a weekly or daily walk, you become not only each other's training partners but also motivator, coach, companion and a source of safety and security.

Complement your walking program with healthy eating habits:

1. Limit the number of times you eat out.
2. Eat breakfast every day.
3. Eat meals (particularly dinner) whenever possible as a family.
4. Turn off the television while you're eating.
5. Limit soda pop intake to 8 ounces (250 milliliters) per week, and fruit juice to 8 ounces per day. Water should be the beverage of choice for thirst quenching, skim milk for mealtimes.
6. Buy only nutritious snack foods to have in the house. If the only available choices are healthy ones, making good choices is easy.
7. Remember that no food item is completely forbidden. Just remember that treats are for special occasions, not for every day.

Choosing a walking partner

If you want to find a walking partner within your community of family and friends, you need to create a mental list of your walking needs. For example, do you want your walking partner to join you for all of your weekly walks? You may enjoy the solitude of your Sunday morning walk but struggle to motivate yourself to get out the door for your midweek walks. Ask yourself if this person is enjoyable to be around, reliable and motivated to walk for exercise. You don't want a walking partner who has a negative attitude, who is perpetually late and who requires continuous cajoling to get out the door. During the chilly days of winter, it will be difficult enough to lace up your own shoes and get moving without having to worry about motivating another person. There will definitely be days when one of you has more interest in walking than the other, but as a general rule, it's a good idea to have comparable fitness levels, goals and enthusiasm.

Walking groups

From women's-only to aging seniors and bereaved widows, there are walking groups for almost every cross section of our society. A walking club isn't for everyone, but many people find it's a great motivator and an easy way to meet people and have fun while exercising.

How to find one in your community

In looking for a suitable walking group you want to first consider your interests and expectations. For example, if you're new to walking for fitness, joining a marathon speed-walking group might not be your best decision. Try to research the various walking groups in your community by going online or by calling the local recreation or community center. Be sure to ask for the group leader's contact information. A quick call or e-mail to the group leader will help you to establish the general demographic of the group as well as the meeting time, location and fitness expectations (distance and speed you will be expected to walk). It's often a good idea to try out a few walking groups in order to figure out the best fit for your fitness goals, personality and schedule.

Start your own walking group

If there isn't a walking group in your community, consider creating your own. Start by posting flyers at your local fitness club, community or seniors' center. You may want to ask your local TV station or community newspaper about advertising in their free community

Sam

Sam is an aging baby boomer who has always thought of himself as an athletic and handsome guy. Successful in most areas of his life, he has a great wife and two healthy and active boys as well as a job as a political strategist, which he loves. A year ago, he began to find the travel and long hours of his job a little demanding and told his wife that he felt his age was starting to slow him down. He said he no longer had the energy or enthusiasm to join his buddies in the weekly hockey match.

Sam was surprised when his wife, Maggie, replied that she had noticed the 15 pounds (6.8 kilograms) he had gained and could understand that the added weight might make him feel lethargic. He knew his waistline had grown, but he didn't think others had noticed. In fact, he assured Maggie that he didn't mind getting a little thicker around the waist—he attributed it to age and a successful career. Maggie disagreed, and said so. A runner who logs 60 miles (100 kilometers) a week, Maggie has the figure of someone half her age. She suggested that Sam join her for a walk after dinner.

Although initially he refused because he thought walking was not "real" exercise, Sam finally agreed. Four nights a week, he and Maggie walk at a brisk pace for almost an hour. It has become "their" time—sometimes they talk about their day, the kids or household issues, but at other times they are silent, enjoying the peacefulness of the night air. Sam has lost the extra weight, is more relaxed and now has more energy than he has had in a long time.

calendars. You want your advertisement and flyers to invite interested walkers to a meeting. Be sure to list your phone number or e-mail address so that interested people can contact you. At the first meeting, encourage everyone to share their ideas, and then as a group decide where, when, how far, how fast and how frequently you will walk. This is a good time to discuss other issues such as what to do if it's raining or snowing, and whether you want to allow folks to use cell phones or wear headphones during the walks.

Motivate your walking group

The following are suggestions for motivating your walking group and ideas for keeping your walks interesting:

- Once a month, meet at a different location for your walk. This way you can explore new parks, trails and neighborhoods.
- Hold the occasional party to celebrate the changing seasons or the anniversary of your walking club. It could be as simple as a post-walk breakfast at a local diner or a potluck dinner at one of the members' homes.
- Invite a guest speaker to attend one of your meetings to discuss an issue that's of interest to your group, for example, the natural habitat in your community or the growing environmental issues facing your local parks and waters.
- Set a group walking goal, such as walking every Sunday morning throughout the winter regardless of snow, wind and rain. Or keep track of the miles you've covered, and once you reach your distance

milestone, celebrate your combined achievement with a night out at the movies.

- Share success stories about achieving personal health and fitness goals.
- Have an expert from a specialty athletic store attend a meeting to talk about proper walking shoes and the best exercise gear for walking in extreme temperatures.

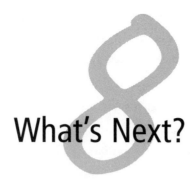

What's Next?

WELL DONE! OVER THE PAST SEVERAL MONTHS YOU HAVE persevered and achieved a new active lifestyle. The walking program you've been following has provided you with a structured plan to get you to a place where you walk almost every day for 20 to 40 minutes or more. For some of you, you're fitter now than ever before. Besides reaping the rewards of improved health, your confidence has skyrocketed. This added confidence and your new-found fitness likely have you wondering, what's next? From destination and charity events to traveling overseas for a walking holiday, the following pages explore a few of the exciting walking opportunities available to you.

Destination Walks

Incorporating a long walk through an unfamiliar community, park or trail every week can add variety to your regular walking program. To find out about great walks in your community, ask at your local tourist information center, go online to research your walking options or purchase a street or trail map at the bookstore. You might consider asking a friend or family member to share in the fun

Make a list of destination walk ideas

1. Tourist places you'd like to visit in your city
2. Parks, tree-lined streets and green spaces to visit in your city
3. Art galleries and museums for indoor walking visits
4. Retail districts for window-shopping walks

of your weekly destination walk and take turns picking new places to visit. Whether you're in phase 2 or phase 4 of the walking program in chapter 3, exploring the sights and sounds of new communities keeps things interesting and is a great motivator for maintaining a regular fitness program. If you're having trouble finding good ideas, consider the following suggestions:

- Make a list of the places you would suggest that a tourist visit in your city and the surrounding communities. Using this list, choose some areas you could make into a destination walk. For example, if your city has a historic site that's of interest, consider including this as part of a longer weekend walk.

- Make a list of all the parks, tree-lined streets and green spaces in your city. When the weather is good, drive or take public transit to one of these destinations and make it part of one of your walks. You could even pack a picnic and eat your lunch among the old-growth trees or flower gardens in your city park.

- If you enjoy visiting art galleries or museums, these are great rainy-day destinations. It may not feel as if you're truly exercising, but you're on your feet and moving. If you want to get in a few more steps, consider walking to your destination, or take public transit and get off at a stop that allows you to walk a few extra blocks.

- If shopping is your thing, you might enjoy an evening of window shopping during a walk through your favorite retail district.

Walking for Fitness

Charity Walks

Signing up for a charity event is not only a way to raise funds and awareness for your favorite charity; it can be a great fitness goal. Never before have there been more charity walks available. Most organizations have detailed Web sites that contain all the information you will need to participate, including registration forms, donation information and event-day details.

Most cities hold walking events throughout the year. They make it easy and convenient to participate. If you recently completed or are about to finish phase 4 of the walking program in chapter 3, you should be ready to sign up for a 3- or 6-mile (5- or 10-kilometer) event soon. If you're partway through phase 4 or an earlier phase of the walking program, consider setting your sights on a specific event and work towards it. Many people find that entering an event gives them the added motivation they need to maintain a regular walking program.

Choose your event

One of the first steps in selecting an event is to establish your goal distance. Charity walks can range anywhere from 3 to 26 miles (5 to 42.2 kilometers) and beyond. Understandably, if you've just completed the 3- or 6-mile (5- or 10-kilometer) walking program in this book, you may want to find an event of similar distance. Regardless of the event distance, many people find that preparing for a specific walk is a great way to stay consistent and on track with their fitness goals. Organized events are also a great way to get out into the

i Get on the computer and do a search using the keywords "charity walks". You'll be amazed at all the possibilities, including tips and helpful support information.

community, see friends and celebrate a healthy lifestyle. If you feel unsure or slightly intimidated about walking a charity event, it's a good idea to watch a local race in your community. You'll be surprised to find that walkers, and runners, come in all shapes, sizes, ages and fitness abilities.

Prepare mentally

You may find that you're a little nervous in the days leading up to your event. Don't worry, this is normal. Even the most seasoned athletes have a few jitters in the days and hours before their event. If you've followed your regular training program to the best of your ability,

Pat

At 65 years of age, Pat has maintained a solid walking program for over 15 years. He initially started walking as a way to lose weight and to better manage the stress he was experiencing from his high-pressure job as a criminal-justice lawyer. At the time, most of his male friends gave him a hard time about walking, suggesting that it wasn't "real" exercise. But after he lost 30 pounds (13.6 kilograms) and became noticeably more relaxed at work, the jokes were replaced with requests to join him on his lunchtime walks.

These days, Pat is retired and regularly joins four friends throughout the week for an hour-long walk. When asked how he continues to motivate himself to maintain his five weekly walks, he says, "I have trained for and completed five half marathons and now I'm training for a 2-day charity walk to end breast cancer. My wife passed away 2 years ago from breast cancer, and raising awareness and money for this cause has become a primary goal. I want to do whatever I can to ensure that if my daughter or any other woman is faced with this dreadful disease they have a better chance of winning the fight than my wife, Ruth."

To train for longer events like the half marathon, Pat follows a 3-month training program that includes three weekly walks and one long walk that he usually does on the weekend. Pat has found following the program—a gradual progression of walking time and distance—allows him to finish the race motivated, happy and free of pain.

you can rest assured that you will have the fitness level required to complete the distance.

Plan ahead

If you take a few minutes to plan ahead, you will be in a better position to enjoy the day of the big event and have fun! The following simple guidelines may help:

The week before

- Check out the map of the course to get a mental picture of the event route.
- Arrange your transportation to and from the event. If it's a large event, you might consider public transit, as parking can be difficult to find on race morning and may increase your pre-race jitters.
- Pick up your race package prior to race day. Besides your race number, which you will pin on your shirt or jacket, a race package usually includes safety pins (for your race number), some event information and your event T-shirt.
- Rest. Don't worry about trying to fit in extra walks in the last few days before the event. Squeezing in more training at this stage will not get you any fitter.

The day before

- Check the weather forecast and plan accordingly. Plan what you will wear for the event as well as a change of clothing for afterward. If it's cold, you'll want to make sure you have lots of warm clothing. Even in warmer temperatures you may feel a slight chill once you cool down after your event.
- Pack a bag for event day. Include your change of

clothes (including footwear). As well, it's a good idea to pack a bottle of water to hydrate after your long walk.

- Pin your race number on your shirt.

The morning of

- Many races have several categories for walkers and runners, so check and double check the start time for your event and make sure you leave yourself plenty of time to get to the start of the race. Also, be sure you know where you will be lining up to start.
- Eat a light meal 2 to 3 hours prior to the start of your event. Be sure to eat something that is familiar to you, such as a bagel and peanut butter, and go easy on the coffee. Now is not the time to try anything new.
- Give yourself 10 to 15 minutes before the start of your event to warm up with some light walking and stretching. You want to keep your heart rate up by moving in one spot before the gun goes off, signaling the start of the event.
- Finally, make sure you visit the restroom before you head to the start line.

The start line

- If there are lots of participants, be sure to walk in a predictable manner. This means walking in a straight line so that faster walkers and runners can easily pass. Sudden movements can cause others to stumble and fall, so be courteous to the people around you. If you are trying to pass someone, make sure that you are a couple of strides ahead before you cut across his or her path.

Walking for Fitness

- Follow the course and avoid cutting corners. After all, doing otherwise is cheating.

After the event
- There will be a finish line to mark the end of your race. Once you cross this line, be sure to keep moving through the finishing chute area. Some events separate women and men, so be sure to take note of which chute is yours.
- Remember to take some time to cool down afterward. It's natural to walk more quickly in the last few miles of your event, so be sure to gradually lower your heart rate with some easy walking and stretching.
- Be sure to rehydrate and refuel. There will be water and refreshments available in the finish area. Help yourself, and enjoy your post-race euphoria!

Walking Holidays: Tours and Hikes

If you're looking for a long-term walking goal, or if you have moved through the first few phases of the walking program, you might want to consider a walking holiday. Vacations are an ideal time to set out on foot to explore this amazing world. Whether you choose a tour company that organizes walking holidays or a self-planned vacation that includes sightseeing on foot, walking is an ideal way to explore cities, discover the magic of ancient ruins or visit a mountainside hideaway.

Organized walking tours

In the last 10 to 15 years, organized walking holidays have become an industry in and of themselves. From

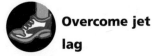

Overcome jet lag

- Assume the local time as soon as possible.
- Try to stick with good nutrition choices, even if it seems easier just to grab something quick and nearby.
- Stay well hydrated. Make a conscious effort to sip water as much as possible.
- Stay away from caffeine of any kind—it will affect your need for sleep.
- Get lots of fresh air—it will make you feel and sleep better.

the Scottish countryside to New York's Chinatown, there are tours for almost every kind of traveler. If you research walking holidays online or ask for information at a travel agency, you will discover that tour companies provide organized walking holidays in most countries. Tours vary from 5 days to 2 weeks, depending on the company and the type of holiday. Most tour operators provide a detailed outline of each tour, including an itinerary for each day, a description of the walks and a list of the sites you will visit along the way. In most cases, travel arrangements upon arrival are organized by the tour company, as well as accommodation and some meals. Most tour companies employ local guides who can show you the hidden charms found off the beaten path and away from the mainstream tourist spots.

Tours are a relaxing way to see the sights of a new city or country. If it's been a while since you've traveled, or if it's your first time traveling outside your country, group tours are also a good way to build your confidence for your voyage. And for women traveling alone, group tours provide the safety of numbers.

Self-planned walking holidays

If an organized walking tour is too costly, overly structured or too limiting for you but you do want to incorporate walking into your travel plans, planning a walking holiday yourself is pretty simple. All you need to do is research areas of interest on the Internet or purchase a guidebook that provides a detailed description of your holiday destination. Using this book, make a list of the parks, trails, museums, galleries and eateries that are of interest. From this list, you can begin to outline a daily itinerary that includes some longer walks along a scenic shoreline or in remote countryside.

Flexibility is one of the most attractive aspects of creating your own walking holiday—you can spend as much or as little time as you want at a given location. You can decide the specific country, city and sights you want to visit. As well, you can plan your own food and accommodation according to your interest and budget. If you decide you want to deviate from your original plans, you can do so with greater ease than if you're with a large group. And traveling alone or with a small group

Harry

Harry is an 85-year-old retired pilot who says he walks for fitness and for his health, physical and mental. He feels so much better when he's had some exercise, especially when it can be outdoors. His love of the outdoors is part of the reason he spends as much time as he can in warmer climates during the winter. Winter weather often makes walking trickier on the trails and he feels a sense of "cabin fever" on days when he doesn't walk, though he does occasionally use the treadmills in his condominium's gym.

Since retirement, Harry has increased his walking time and intensity, especially when he's not taking classes in aerobics, line dancing or water aerobics. He's fortunate that the city where he lives, Mississauga, has an excellent trail system, as all new developments are required to have a link to the trails. Harry says, "It will take a long time for me to explore the Mississauga trails, some of which follow creeks, rivers or the shore of Lake Ontario."

Harry has a son living in Antigua, where he's had beautiful walks, and another son in Melbourne, Australia, a city that provides well for walkers, runners and cyclists. On a recent visit to Melbourne, Harry took a long walk along the bay, through a park with colorful birds (and a mysterious animal that turned out to be a possum) and finally along many little lanes lined with charming Edwardian buildings.

Harry says, "As long as there is beauty to see—a rose growing in someone's garden, a butterfly, wildflowers—my walk is interesting."

If you do want to find the time to walk while you're away, try a morning walk. This is a great time to do a little sightseeing on foot—no doubt you'll seek out a nice quiet neighborhood or park that you wouldn't have discovered otherwise. If your guidebook or fellow travelers don't turn up any options, hotel staff members are always a good resource.

often increases the likelihood of meeting interesting locals and exploring the less touristy spots. As long as you do the research beforehand and speak with some of the locals upon your arrival, you will easily be able to incorporate walking and sightseeing into your next holiday.

Nordic Walking

If you're able to walk most days for 20 to 40 minutes and you're looking for a great cardiovascular activity that works your entire body, you might want to try Nordic walking. This sport originated in Finland as a summer cross-training activity for skiers, since it is similar to cross-country skiing, only without the snow. Using specially designed poles similar to those used for cross-country skiing, Nordic walkers stride along trails and roads while using a technique that engages the upper body and back as well as the lower portion of the body. The growing popularity of Nordic walking can be attributed to the incredible workout that it provides.

Essentially, each time you swing your arm forward, you must plant your pole into the ground behind you in order to push off or "propel" yourself forward. This motion engages your arms, core muscles (stomach and lower back), shoulders and upper back. It takes a little time to get comfortable with the poling motion, but most people find that with correct instruction they are comfortable within an hour or so of practicing the new motion. When it's done properly, Nordic walking gives almost 95 percent of the body's muscles a workout. As well, the poling action as well as the actual pole materials absorb a significant portion of the impact. With a good Nordic pole, there is a rubber "paw" on the tip that also helps to absorb some of the impact. All of this means fewer demands on the muscles and ligaments, making it an ideal activity for people with knee problems, pregnant woman and those looking for a different aerobic exercise. If you're interested in learning more about Nordic walking, many community and fitness centers now offer classes, or you can purchase poles and a how-to DVD or book at most major athletic or cross-country ski stores.

Hiking and Trekking

Hiking, trekking and trail walking are all terms used to describe a form of walking that takes place outside with the purpose of exercising and exploring the natural beauty of the outdoors. Hiking is usually done on park trails or in relatively unspoiled wilderness parks.

To find out about trails in your community, or if you want to do some hiking while traveling on holidays, many hiking guidebooks and Web sites provide detailed information on regional treks. Once you arrive at your hiking destination, there is usually a sign posted at the trail entrance listing the length and difficulty of the various trails. Keep in mind that the posted distance is typically one-way, so you will need to gauge your speed and endurance appropriately. As well, most trails are assigned a grade according to the level of difficulty. Total distance, hilliness, terrain and altitude are factors that determine whether a hike is easy or exceptionally difficult. If you're new to hiking, it's a good idea to start

Are you hiking ready?

- You have completed the lifestyle walking program and can walk for 1 hour a few times a week.
- You regularly incorporate hills into your walk sessions.
- You can climb 3 to 4 flights of stairs without being winded.
- You can step on and off sidewalk curbs without falling.
- You don't have any lingering pains or injuries.
- You don't have any health problems that require you to stay close to a hospital.

with beginner hikes to build your strength and confidence before attempting a more difficult hike.

One final note: Hiking is a great way to get some exercise and explore the natural beauty of the outdoors, but you want to make sure that safety is at the top of your priority list. This means always telling someone where you're hiking and how long you will be away, knowing the area and making sure you are dressed appropriately. Also, be sure to carry extra water, a flashlight, matches, first aid kit and food in the event that your hike takes you longer than planned.

Organized hikes and trekking groups

Hiking and trail-walking groups exist in most communities. If you live in a community where there are surrounding hiking trails, or if you're planning to visit a wilderness region on your next holiday, you might consider inquiring with the local community or seniors' center for information on trail-walking groups. In North Vancouver, British Columbia, for example, the Trail Trekkers are a group that has been actively exploring the North Shore mountains for more than 20 years. As long as you can easily walk for 2 hours, the Trail Trekkers welcome hikers to join any of their numerous weekly treks. If you're interested in hiking but you've never done it before, joining a group is a safe way to increase your confidence to explore the wilderness, and it's a good way to meet people who share the same passion.

Speed Walking

If you've progressed to phase 3 of the walking program and you want to improve your fitness, increase your calorie burn rate and try something new, you may want to try speed walking. Also referred to as power walking, fitness walking, health walking or striding, speed walking is a great fitness exercise. With less jarring of the muscles and bones than in running, speed walking is an ideal way to increase strength and endurance with little risk of injury. It's basically fast walking without any jogging or running.

If you want to pick up your walking pace and become a speed walker, first consult your physician about your new fitness goals. You want to be certain that there aren't any health risks associated with increasing your level of exertion. After you've received the okay from your doctor, you can teach yourself to speed walk: simply increase your walking pace and focus on a good arm swing. Your arm swing is in keeping with your foot pace: one foot must be on the ground at all times, and your stride is usually quicker and longer than when you're walking at a leisurely pace. If you want to master the correct technique, there are speed-walking clinics offered at health clubs, community centers and through walking groups. Or you can pick up a book or video that outlines the specifics of speed walking.

Race Walking

You might have seen race-walking events on television or at a track meet and wondered what those seemingly strange people were doing with their exaggerated hip rotation and upward carriage. What you may not realize is that race walking is considered one of the first athletic endeavors, with races dating back to the 17th and 18th centuries. Since 1908, race walking has been an official Olympic sport, with women's events added in 1992.

Not merely fast walking, race walking requires a specific technique that takes time to perfect. Unlike running, your body cannot become airborne, which means that one foot must remain on the ground at all times. Besides this, race walking requires that the heel of the foot touch the ground first and that the supporting leg not bend and the knee stay locked from the time the foot is first planted on the ground to when the leg moves under your body. The arm swing of a race walker

Bruce

Bruce is a fit 79-year-old who has been active for most of his life. In his earlier years, he enjoyed playing volleyball, weight training and cross-country skiing. About 10 years ago, he realized that if he wanted to stay active as he aged, he would have to search out a different exercise program. At the time, his wife, Cynthia, was already an avid walker, so it seemed an easy decision to join her on some of her walks.

Bruce and Cynthia have organized several of their own walking holidays, including a walk that took them from the North Sea to the Irish Sea as well as to Hadrian's Wall in Newcastle, United Kingdom. While on holiday, they often walk 12 miles (20 kilometers) per day for up to 10 consecutive days. In preparation for these walking holidays, they increase the distance and the intensity of their walks about 6 months before the start of their trip. Their training includes about three walks per week, two of which Bruce does by completing his errands on foot. He finds walking to the grocery store and to the bank great ways to stay on track with his fitness program and to use his car a little less, which is good for the environment.

An essential part of Bruce and Cynthia's preparation for their walking holidays is one long walk a week. Their long walks are usually 12 to 16 miles (20 to 25 kilometers), and they try to incorporate winding paths or steep hills in an effort to mirror the terrain of their next walking tour.

is strenuous and accentuated. Because the supporting leg must remain unbent at all times, the torso and pelvic rotation can be considered the sport's most distinguishing characteristics.

If you're interested in learning how to race walk, some walking groups and sport stores offer clinics. Or you can purchase a book or video that outlines in detail the specific race-walking techniques. But just as with speed walking, you want to be sure to check with your family physician for medical clearance before embarking on a race-walking program.

Running

If you've completed the final phases of the walking program and are looking for another challenge, you might want to try a learn-to-run program. *The Beginning Runner's Handbook* includes tips and advice for new runners as well as a gradual and progressive walk/run program that intersperses walking with running.

You did it! You set your sights on improving your fitness, and you did it. Congratulations! Becoming a person who walks regularly for exercise is no easy feat—be sure to take some time to celebrate your amazing achievement. Over time you may want to refer to this book for motivation or advice; after all, an active lifestyle is a life-long pursuit, but it's well worth the effort. Good luck, and enjoy your newfound fitness!

Appendix A

Stretching Exercises

Here are some stretches for the major muscle groups used in walking. Use them as a guide to building your own routine. It's a good idea to work systematically from the calves up to the shoulders (or vice versa).

Before stretching, always start with 5 to 10 minutes of easy walking to warm your muscles. Then move into your pre-training stretching exercises. Hold each position (no bouncing) for approximately 30 seconds. Your stretching routine should take no more than 10 to 12 minutes.

After your workout, use the same stretches to cool down. If you wish to work on increasing your flexibility, hold the stretches for longer—anywhere from 30 seconds to 3 minutes—and repeat each stretch 2 to 3 times. Pay particular attention to the areas that you feel are the tightest; in walkers, these are usually the lower back, hamstrings and calves.

Calf

1. Stand facing a wall, an arm's length plus 6 inches (15 centimeters) away.
2. Place your right foot forward, halfway to the wall, and bend your right knee while keeping your left leg straight.

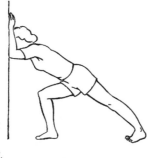

3. Lean into the wall, pushing your left heel into the floor while keeping your head, neck, spine, pelvis and left leg in a straight line.
4. Hold the stretch for 30 seconds and relax.
5. Repeat, starting with your left leg forward.

Hamstring

This exercise requires a doorway.

1. Lie flat on your back, through a doorway, positioning your hips slightly in front of the door frame, with the inside of your lower right thigh against one side of the frame.

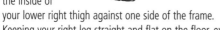

2. Keeping your right leg straight and flat on the floor, exhale and raise your left leg until your heel rests against the door frame. Do not bend your left knee.
3. Hold the stretch for 30 seconds and relax.
4. To increase the stretch, slide your buttocks closer to the door frame, or lift the leg away from the frame to create a right angle.
5. Repeat with your right leg raised.

Iliotibial Band

1. Stand with your left side toward a wall, an arm's length away, feet together.
2. Extend your left arm sideways at shoulder height so the flat of your hand is against the wall and you are leaning toward it.

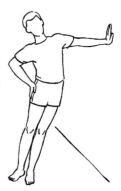

3. Exhale, and push your left hip in toward the wall until you feel the stretch down the outside of your left hip/thigh.
4. Hold the stretch for 30 seconds and relax.
5. Repeat on the right side.

Quadriceps

Avoid this exercise if it causes pain in the knee joint.

1. Stand tall, facing a wall, an arm's length away; place your right hand against the wall for balance and support.
2. Bend your left leg at the knee and raise the foot behind you until you can grasp it with your left hand.

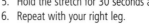

3. Slightly bend your right leg at the knee and be sure to keep your lower back straight.
4. Keeping the knees together, pull your left heel toward your buttock.
5. Hold the stretch for 30 seconds and relax.
6. Repeat with your right leg.

Groin

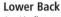

1. Sit upright on the floor, with your back against a wall.
2. Bend your knees up, then let them fall to the sides, with the soles of your feet facing each other.
3. Grasp your ankles with both hands and pull your heels toward your buttocks.
4. Rest your elbows on the inside of your thighs.
5. Slowly push your knees toward the floor until you feel the stretch in your groin.
6. Hold the stretch for 30 seconds and relax.

Hip Flexor

For those who are unable to kneel, this exercise can be done while sitting on the edge of a chair and assuming the same position as illustrated but without the knee touching the ground.

1. Stand with your feet hip-width apart.
2. Flexing your right knee, slowly lower your body toward the ground, finishing with your left knee touching the floor and your right heel flat on the floor.
3. Rest your hands just above the right knee, and keep that knee bent at no more than a right angle.
4. For some, getting into this position will be enough. If you wish to increase the stretch, exhale while pushing your left hip forward and increasing the stretch on the left side.
5. Hold the stretch for 30 seconds and relax.
6. Repeat with your left foot forward.

Gluteal

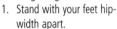

1. Lie flat on your back with your legs straight and arms out to the sides.
2. Bend the left knee and raise it toward your chest, grasping your knee or thigh with your right hand.
3. Keep your head, shoulders and elbows flat on the floor.
4. Exhale as you pull your knee across your body toward the floor.
5. Hold the stretch for 30 seconds and relax.
6. For a deeper stretch, straighten the top leg.
7. Repeat with the right leg.

Lower Back

1. Lie flat on your back with your knees bent to form a right angle and your arms out to the sides.
2. Exhale, and slowly lower both knees to the left side.
3. Keep your elbows, head and shoulders flat on the floor.
4. Hold the stretch for 30 seconds and relax.
5. Repeat on the right side.

Lower Back

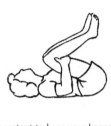

1. Lie flat on your back with your legs straight out.
2. Bend your knees and slide your heels toward your buttocks.
3. Using both hands, grasp behind your knees. (It's not important to keep your knees together—they should be comfortable.)
4. Exhale, pulling your knees toward your chest and slowly lifting your hips from the floor, while keeping your head and shoulders on the floor.
5. Hold the stretch for 30 seconds and relax.

Chest and Shoulder Stretch

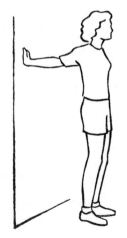

1. Stand with your right arm straight and your right hand pressed against a wall behind you.
2. Walk your feet around so the toes point away from the wall.
3. With your right hand still resting against the wall, twist your hips and shoulders away from the wall, until you feel a slight stretch in the chest and shoulder.
4. Hold the stretch for 30 seconds and relax.
5. Repeat with left arm.

Appendix B

(http://www.lcsd.gov.hk/en/forms/parq.pdf)

Physical Activity Readiness
Questionnaire - PAR-Q
(revised - 2006)

PAR-Q & YOU

(A Questionnaire for People Aged 15 to 69)

Regular physical activity is fun and healthy, and increasingly more people are starting to become more active every day. Being more active is very safe for most people. However, some people should check with their doctor before they start becoming much more physically active.

If you are planning to become much more physically active than you are now, start by answering the seven questions in the box below. If you are between the ages of 15 and 69, the PAR-Q will tell you if you should check with your doctor before you start. If you are over 69 years of age, and you are not used to being very active, check with your doctor.

Common sense is your best guide when you answer these questions. Please read the questions carefully and answer each one honestly : Check YES or NO.

YES	NO		
☐	☐	1.	Has your doctor ever said that you have a heart condition and that you should only do physical activity recommended by a doctor?
☐	☐	2.	Do you feel pain in your chest when you do physical activity?
☐	☐	3.	In the past month, have you had chest pain when you were not doing physical activity?
☐	☐	4.	Do you lose your balance because of dizziness or do you ever lose consciousness?
☐	☐	5.	Do you have a bone or joint problem (for example, back, knee or hip) that could be made worse by a change in your physical activity?
☐	☐	6.	Is your doctor currently prescribing drugs (for example, water pills) for your blood pressure or heart condition?
☐	☐	7.	Do you know of any other reason why you should not do physical activity?

If

you

answered

YES to one or more questions

Talk with your doctor by phone or in person BEFORE you start becoming much more physically active or BEFORE you have a fitness appraisal. Tell your doctor about the PAR-Q and which questions you answered YES.

- You may be able to do any activity you want - as long as you start slowly and build up gradually. Or, you may need to restrict your activities to those which are safe for you. Talk with your doctor about the kinds of activities you wish to participate in and follow his/her advice.
- Find out which community programs are safe and helpful for you.

NO to all questions

If you answered NO honestly to all PAR-Q questions, you can be reasonably sure that you can :
- start becoming much more physically active - begin slowly and build up gradually. This is the safest and easiest way to go.
- take part in a fitness appraisal - this is an excellent way to determine your basic fitness so that you can plan the best way for you to live actively. It is also highly recommended that you have your blood pressure evaluated. If your reading is over 144/94, talk with your doctor before you start becoming much more physically active.

→ **DELAY BECOMING MUCH MORE ACTIVE:**
- if you are not feeling well because of a temporary illness such as a cold or a fever - wait until you feel better; or
- if you are or may be pregnant - talk to your doctor before you start becoming more active.

Please note: If your health changes so that you then answer "YES" to any of the above questions, tell your fitness or health professional. Ask whether you should change your physical activity plan.

Informed Use of the PAR-Q: The Canadian Society for Exercise Physiology, Health Canada, and their agents assume no liability for persons who undertake physical activity, and if in doubt after completing this questionnaire, consult your doctor prior to physical activity.

No changes permitted. You are encouraged to photocopy the PAR-Q but only if you use the entire form.

NOTE: If the PAR-Q is being given to a person before he or she participates in a physical activity program or a fitness appraisal, this section may be used for l
egal or administrative purposes.
"I have read, understood and completed this questionnaire. Any questions I had were answered to my full satisfaction."

Name _____   Identity Document No. _____

Signature _____   Date _____

Signature of Parent or Guardian _____   Witness _____
(for participants under the age of majority)

Note: The information provided on this form will only be used for the application for use of Leisure and Cultural Services Department's Fitness Rooms and enrolment of recreation and sports activities. For correction of or access to personal data collected by means of this form, please contact staff of the enrollment counter/district.
This physical activity clearance is valid for a maximum of 12 months from the date it is completed and becomes invalid if your condition changes so that you would answer YES to any of the seven questions.

©Canadian Society for Exercise Physiology   Supported by : Health Canada

Appendix C

Shoe-shopping Tips

A well-trained sales person can identify any obvious anomalies in your gait or foot mechanics, determine the proper size and width of your foot and provide you with some meaningful footwear options. These options should be tailored to your specific needs. After the salesperson watches you walk in each pair of shoes and guides you appropriately, your final choice should come down to fit and comfort. Remember the following points when purchasing your walking shoes:

- Many people have problems with their walking gait that, if ignored, can result in problems. For example, when your foot impacts the ground on the lateral (outer) part of the heel and then rolls inward towards the arch, you are *pronating*. In most cases, this motion is efficient, but if it's done excessively it can cause problems in your ankles, knees and even your lower back.

- When you go to a specialty shoe or athletic-outfitting store to purchase your walking shoes, be sure to speak with a trained salesperson so that he or she can identify whether you pronate or supinate. *Supinators* are folks whose feet roll outward.

- If you do have one of these gait problems, you will want to purchase a shoe that is specifically designed to correct pronation or supination.

- If you are blessed with good feet and sound biomechanics, you can usually walk injury free in almost any shoe. From the casual style of a well-made walking shoe to the athletic design of a good sneaker, the choice will be mostly a matter of fit and comfort.

- The more stylish walking shoe is a common choice for those who walk a great deal at work or on holiday. But finding a so-called "brown" shoe with the key technical features demanded by the problematic foot can be difficult. Therefore, those with problem feet will be served better by purchasing a well-cushioned athletic walking or running shoe.

- If you have bunions or a history of pain at the ball of your foot (metatarsalgia) due to neuromas or arthritis, you may find relief in a stiffer, more rocker-soled shoe. A rocker-soled shoe means there is a permanent modification to the outer sole of the shoe. The slight U-shaped sole is designed to increase the support available through the midfoot.

- Even though the heel strike position and impact forces differ between walking and running, your final choice of shoe should be based on your biomechanics and two final criteria... *fit* and *comfort.*

- Keep in mind that shoes don't last forever! The rule of thumb is that after 500 miles (805 kilometers) of wear, the cushioning as well as the support of the shoe has been compromised. To put it in perspective: if you walk 3 times a week for an hour at a time, that's about 10 miles (16 kilometers) a week, or 40 miles (64 kilometers) a month... or about 500 miles (800 kilometers) a year.

- At 500 miles, the shoe will feel flat and unsupportive compared with a new model. Old and wornout shoes can cause a slight ache in the arch of your foot or a tweak in your knee.

Appendix D

InTraining to Walk 10 Km Program

Is this YOU? "I have worked through phase 4 and would enjoy challenging myself further." Or "I am already an avid walker, able to walk 30 to 60 minutes almost every day, depending on how I feel."

Goal: To prepare for some longer hikes or walks up of to 3 hours, a distance of about 10 kilometers.

Week 1		
Session 1	44 minutes	Warm-up: A slow and easy walk for 10 minutes.
		A 3-minute brisk walk followed by a 2-minute slow and easy recovery walk.
		A 2-minute brisk walk followed by a 2-minute recovery walk.
		A 1-minute brisk walk followed by a 2-minute recovery walk.
		Repeat this combination 2 times.
		Cool-down: A slow and easy walk for 10 minutes.
Session 2	30 minutes	Warm-up: A slow and easy walk for 5 minutes.
		Walk for 20 minutes.
		Cool-down: A slow and easy walk for 5 minutes.
Session 3	35 minutes	Warm-up: A slow and easy walk for 5 minutes.
		Walk for 25 minutes.
		Cool-down: A slow and easy walk for 5 minutes.

Week 2		
Session 1	40 minutes	Warm-up: A slow and easy walk for 10 minutes.
		A 2-minute brisk walk followed by a 2-minute slow and easy recovery walk.
		Repeat this combination 5 times.
		Cool-down: A slow and easy walk for 10 minutes.
Session 2	30 minutes	Warm-up: A slow and easy walk for 5 minutes.
		Walk for 20 minutes.
		Cool-down: A slow and easy walk for 5 minutes.

Session 3	40 minutes	Warm-up: A slow and easy walk for 5 minutes.
		Walk for 30 minutes.
		Cool-down: A slow and easy walk for 5 minutes.

Week 3

Session 1	54 minutes	Warm-up: A slow and easy walk for 15 minutes.
		A 1-minute brisk walk followed by a 2-minute slow and easy recovery walk.
		Repeat this combination 8 times.
		Cool-down: A slow and easy walk for 15 minutes.

Session 2	40 minutes	Warm-up: A slow and easy walk for 5 minutes.
		Walk for 30 minutes.
		Cool-down: A slow and easy walk for 5 minutes.

Session 3	50 minutes	Warm-up: A slow and easy walk for 5 minutes.
		Walk for 40 minutes.
		Cool-down: A slow and easy walk for 5 minutes.

Week 4: Easy Recovery Week

Session 1	40 minutes	Warm-up: A slow and easy walk for 10 minutes.
		An easy 20-minute walk.
		Cool-down: A slow and easy walk for 10 minutes.

Session 2	30 minutes	Warm-up: A slow and easy walk for 5 minutes.
		Walk for 20 minutes.
		Cool-down: A slow and easy walk for 5 minutes.

Session 3	40 minutes	Warm-up: A slow and easy walk for 5 minutes.
		Walk for 30 minutes.
		Cool-down: A slow and easy walk for 5 minutes.

Week 5

Session 1	51 minutes	Warm-up: A slow and easy walk for 15 minutes.
		A 5-minute brisk walk followed by a 2-minute slow and easy recovery walk.
		Repeat this combination 3 times.
		Cool-down: A slow and easy walk for 15 minutes.

Session 2	40 minutes	Warm-up: A slow and easy walk for 5 minutes.
		Walk for 30 minutes.
		Cool-down: A slow and easy walk for 5 minutes.
Session 3	50 minutes	Warm-up: A slow and easy walk for 5 minutes.
		Walk for 40 minutes.
		Cool-down: A slow and easy walk for 5 minutes.

Week 6

Session 1	66 minutes	Warm-up: A slow and easy walk for 15 minutes.
		A 3-minute brisk walk followed by a 2-minute slow and easy recovery walk.
		A 2-minute brisk walk followed by a 2-minute slow and easy recovery walk.
		A 1-minute brisk walk followed by a 2-minute slow and easy recovery walk.
		Repeat this combination 3 times.
		Cool-down: A slow and easy walk for 15 minutes.
Session 2	40 minutes	Warm-up: A slow and easy walk for 5 minutes.
		Walk for 30 minutes.
		Cool-down: A slow and easy walk for 5 minutes.
Session 3	60 minutes	Warm-up: A slow and easy walk for 5 minutes.
		Walk for 50 minutes.
		Cool-down: A slow and easy walk for 5 minutes.

Week 7: Over Halfway!

Session 1	60 minutes or 5 km	Warm-up: A slow and easy walk for 5 minutes.
		Walk for 60 minutes, or about 5 kilometers.
		Cool-down: A slow and easy walk for 5 minutes.
Session 2	50 minutes	Warm-up: A slow and easy walk for 5 minutes.
		Walk for 40 minutes.
		Cool-down: A slow and easy walk for 5 minutes.
Session 3	70 minutes	Warm-up: A slow and easy walk for 5 minutes.
		Walk for 60 minutes.
		Cool-down: A slow and easy walk for 5 minutes.

Week 8: Easy Recovery Week

Session 1   70 minutes   Warm-up: A slow and easy walk for 5 minutes.

Walk for 60 minutes.

Cool-down: A slow and easy walk for 5 minutes.

Session 2   30 minutes   Warm-up: A slow and easy walk for 5 minutes.

Walk for 20 minutes.

Cool-down: A slow and easy walk for 5 minutes.

Session 3   40 minutes   Warm-up: A slow and easy walk for 5 minutes.

Walk for 30 minutes.

Cool-down: A slow and easy walk for 5 minutes.

Week 9

Session 1   80 minutes   Warm-up: A slow and easy walk for 15 minutes.

A 5-minute brisk walk followed by a 2-minute slow and easy recovery walk.

A 4-minute brisk walk followed by a 2-minute recovery walk.

A 3-minute brisk walk followed by a 2-minute recovery walk.

A 2-minute brisk walk followed by a 2-minute recovery walk.

A 1-minute brisk walk followed by a 2-minute recovery walk.

Repeat this combination 2 times.

Cool-down: A slow and easy walk for 15 minutes.

Session 2   50 minutes   Warm-up: A slow and easy walk for 5 minutes.

Walk for 40 minutes.

Cool-down: A slow and easy walk for 5 minutes.

Session 3   70 minutes   Warm-up: A slow and easy walk for 5 minutes.

Walk for 60 minutes.

Cool-down: A slow and easy walk for 5 minutes.

Week 10

Session 1   80 minutes   Warm-up: A slow and easy walk for 20 minutes.

A 2-minute brisk walk followed by a 2-minute slow and easy recovery walk.

Repeat this combination 10 times.

Cool-down: A slow and easy walk for 20 minutes.

Session 2	50 minutes	Warm-up: A slow and easy walk for 5 minutes.
		Walk for 40 minutes.
		Cool-down: A slow and easy walk for 5 minutes.
Session 3	80 minutes	Warm-up: A slow and easy walk for 5 minutes.
		Walk for 70 minutes.
		Cool-down: A slow and easy walk for 5 minutes.

Week 11

Session 1	90 minutes	Warm-up: A slow and easy walk for 15 minutes.
		Find a hill that has an incline of about 25 degrees:
		A 1-minute brisk walk uphill followed by a walk down the hill at a slow and easy recovery walk pace.
		Repeat this combination 8 times.
		A 30-second brisk walk uphill followed by a walk down the hill at a slow and easy recovery pace.
		Repeat this combination 8 times.
		No hill option:
		A 2-minute brisk walk followed by a 2-minute slow and easy recovery walk. Repeat this combination 6 times.
		A 1-minute brisk walk followed by a 2-minute slow and easy recovery walk. Repeat this combination 6 times.
		Cool-down: A slow and easy walk for 15 minutes.
Session 2	50 minutes	Warm-up: A slow and easy walk for 5 minutes.
		Walk for 40 minutes.
		Cool-down: A slow and easy walk for 5 minutes.
Session 3	70 minutes	Warm-up: A slow and easy walk for 5 minutes.
		Walk for 60 minutes.
		Cool-down: A slow and easy walk for 5 minutes.

Week 12: Easy Recovery Week

Session 1	90 minutes	Warm-up: A slow and easy walk for 5 minutes.
		Walk for 80 minutes.
		Cool-down: A slow and easy walk for 5 minutes.

Session 2	50 minutes	Warm-up: A slow and easy walk for 5 minutes. Walk for 40 minutes.
Session 3	75 minutes	Warm-up: A slow and easy walk for 5 minutes. Walk for 65 minutes. Cool-down: A slow and easy walk for 5 minutes.

Week 13: This is It!

Session 1	44 minutes	Warm-up: A slow and easy walk for 10 minutes. A 3-minute brisk walk followed by a 2-minute slow and easy recovery walk. A 2-minute brisk walk followed by a 2-minute recovery walk. A 1-minute brisk walk followed by a 2-minute recovery walk. Repeat this combination 2 times. Cool-down: A slow and easy walk for 10 minutes.
Session 2	40 minutes	Warm-up: A slow and easy walk for 5 minutes. Walk for 30 minutes. Cool-down: A slow and easy walk for 5 minutes.
Session 3		Event-Day 10 kilometers: Have fun, and take care not to start out too quickly.

Congratulations!

Index

feet. *See* gait and gait problems; shoes; *specific injuries and diseases*; walking technique

Finegood, Diane, 82, 83

first aid. *See* injuries

fitness. *See* cardiovascular fitness

flexibility, 18–20, 48, 94, 106, 145–46. *See also* stretching

fluid balance. *See* hydration

footwear, 41, 101, 106, 148–49

fractures, 15, 16–17

Friedman, Sandy, on weight control, 20

gait and gait problems, 41, 100, 148. *See also* walking technique

gestational diabetes, 115

Gibson, Jennifer, on nutrition, 73, 74, 77, 81, 86

goals, 59, 61–65, 67. *See also* motivation

Greenberg, Jerrold S., on components of health, 55–56

health walking, 141

heart health: angina, 16; body weight and, 82–83; coronary heart disease, 15, 16, 71; diet and, 74–75; exercise and, 14; heart attacks, 16; medical evaluation of, 28. *See also* cardiovascular fitness

hiking and trekking, 139–40

hills, 51–52, 140, 154

hip fractures, 15

hydration, 79, 83–86, 88; on charity walks, 135; dehydration, 84, 98, 103–4; in hot weather, 47; overhydration, 86; during pregnancy, 115

hyponatremia, 86

icing of injuries, 112

illness and walking, 14, 21, 84, 147

injuries: assessment of, 99–101; athlete's foot, 103; avoiding, 36, 95–96, 97–99, 104–6, 109–11; blisters, 102–3; and body changes from exercise, 93–95, 96–97; chafing, 101–2; flexibility and, 19;

fractures, 15, 16–17; muscle cramps and stitches, 103–4; from overuse, 95–96; plantar fasciitis, 106; and shoe choice, 148–49; sore knees, 108; sprained ankle, 107–8; treating at home, 102, 106, 107–8, 111–12. *See also* pain

injury awareness scale, 100

jet lag, 136

journals. *See* logbooks

Joy, Liz, on pregnant walkers, 114–15

knee pain, 100, 101, 108, 139

Lifestyle Walking Program, 45–46

lights, for visibility, 39

Liu-Ambrose, Teresa, on bone health, 17

logbooks, 70, 96, 98

lubricants, 105

mall walking, 24, 34, 35

massage, 104, 108

medical care: checkups for pregnant walkers, 116; checkups for speed and race walking, 141, 143; checkups for walking program, 27–28, 29–30, 99; injuries and, 104, 106, 108, 109; sport medicine podiatrists, 100

menopause, 14–15

mental alertness, and exercise, 94

metatarsalgia, 149

moderation, in exercise, 28, 39, 115

mood, effect of exercise on, 14–15, 17–18, 58

Moore, Phil, on walking shoes, 41

motivation: for behavioral change, 66; for charity walks, 132; for children, 121; tips for improvement, 53–54, 58–61, 67–69; walking partners and groups, 122, 124, 126–27. *See also* goals

muscle cramps, 103–4

muscle soreness and stiffness, 29–30, 94, 96–97

muscle strength, 14, 19, 94, 96–97. *See also* core strength

music for walking, 25, 40–41

neuropathy, injury risks, 98–99

Nordic walking, 138–39

NSAIDS (non-steroid anti-inflammatory drugs), 99

nutrition: before and after charity walks, 134; childhood obesity, 118–19; 80/20 rule, 76, 87; exercise and, 91; fluids, 83–86; food groups, 74–75; meal planning and portions, 74–76, 78–80, 89–90, 123; during pregnancy, 115; tips for healthy eating, 86–88; for weight control, 76–78, 81–83, 118–19. *See also* hydration

obesity. *See* weight control

optimism, 66–67, 71

osteoporosis. *See* bone density

overhydration, 86

overuse injuries, 95–96

pace, 29, 49, 50–51, 97

pain: abdominal stitches, 104; appropriate response to, 95–96; assessment of, 99–101; in back, neck and shoulders, 108–9, 146; drugs for, with diabetes, 99; in knees, 100, 101, 108, 139; "no pain, no gain", 97; plantar fasciitis, 106; and shoe choice, 148–49; sprained ankle, 107–8; symptom of injury, 111. *See also* injuries

Pargman, David, on components of health, 55–56

PAR-Q (Physical Activity Readiness Questionnaire), 28, 147

patience, 13, 39, 52–53

pedometers, 69, 70–71

peripheral vascular disease, 94

Physical Activity Readiness Questionnaire (PAR-Q), 28, 147

places to walk, 34–39

plantar fasciitis, 106

posture, 29, 50, 108–9, 116–17, 138–39

power walking, 141

pregnant walkers, 114–16, 117

Prochaska, James O., 66

pronation, 148

psychology of exercise. *See* goals; motivation

race walking, 51, 141–43

relaxation, 50, 101, 109

rest: injuries and, 111–12; pregnancy and, 115, 116; for recovery and fitness gains, 28, 29, 30, 93–94, 97–98. *See also* walking programs

RICE, 111–12

Rochon, Diana, 59, 108

"runner's high", 56

running, 41, 143

safety, 37–38, 39–41, 42, 44, 140

scheduling meals and snacks, 78–80

scheduling walking time: on calendar, 114; for consistency, 15, 53–54, 56, 57; in daily routines, 33–34; rest days, 97–98; walking partners and groups, 123

Sedgwick, Whitney, 61, 65, 68

self-esteem and weight control, 20–21

shoes, 41, 101, 106, 148–49

sleep, 18, 51, 77, 136

Smith, Trent, on childhood obesity, 118–19, 121

smoking, 16, 17, 20

socializing and walking: with family, 113–22; indoors and outdoors, 37; for motivation and enjoyment, 23–24, 53, 60–61; walking partners and groups, 24, 33, 122, 123–27. *See also* families

speed walking, 141

sport drinks, 86

sport medicine podiatrists, 100. *See also* medical care

sport watches, 32

sprained ankles, 107–8

stitches (abdominal pain), 104

stress management, 16, 17–18, 57

stretching, 18–20, 103–4, 145–46

striding, 141

supination, 148

surfaces for walking, 37, 38–39, 110, 116–17

Suzuki, David, on walking as transportation, 22–23

talk test, 49, 97

technique for walking. *See* walking technique

television: and childhood obesity, 118, 119, 121; and nutrition, 88, 123; while exercising, 36

thirst. *See* hydration

tours, 135–38

tracks, 37, 38–39

traffic, safety in, 39, 42, 44

Trail Trekkers, 140

training programs. *See* walking programs

transportation, walking for, 21–23

treadmills, 36

waist circumference, 81–83

walking clinics, 48

walking partners and groups. *See* socializing and walking

walking programs: for charity walks, 131–32, 133; Lifestyle Walking Program, 45–46; planning and starting, 13, 27–28, 30–32, 52–53; for pregnant walkers, 116; principles of, 43–44; for 10 km walks, 150–55

walking technique, 49–51, 58, 100–101, 138–39, 141, 142–43

walking tours and holidays, 135–38, 140, 142

warming up, 47, 134, 150–55. *See also* walking programs

water intake. *See* hydration

weather: dressing for, 51, 105–6, 133; heat, 24, 47; hydration, 47, 84–85; indoor vs. outdoor walking, 35; rain, 53; sun protection, 48; winter, 38

weight control: assessing need for, 81–83; in children, 118–19, 121–22; decreases stress on joints, 94; diet and, 19, 76–78, 81–83, 90, 118–19; obesity and injuries, 98; pedometers and, 71; thinness and health, 20; walking for, 15, 19, 20–21, 90

when to walk. *See* scheduling walking time

where to walk, 34–39

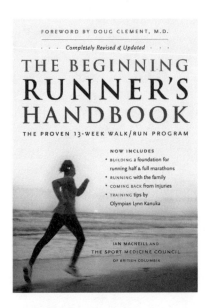
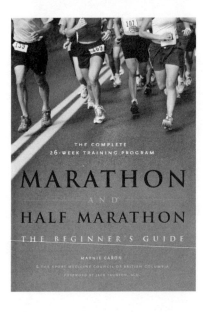